GENETIC AND ENVIRONMENTAL FACTORS
IN HUMAN ABILITY

AF878313

GENETIC AND ENVIRONMENTAL FACTORS IN HUMAN ABILITY

A Symposium held by the Eugenics Society in September–October 1965

Edited by

J. E. MEADE
Professor of Political Economy
University of Cambridge

A. S. PARKES
Mary Marshal Professor of the Physiology of Reproduction
University of Cambridge

Springer-Science+Business Media, B.V.

1966

Library of Congress Catalog Card Number
66-29858

ISBN 978-1-4899-6236-2 ISBN 978-1-4899-6499-1 (eBook)
DOI 10.1007/978-1-4899-6499-1

© 1966 Springer Science+Business Media Dordrecht
Originally published by The Eugenics Society in 1966.
Softcover reprint of the hardcover 1st edition 1966

EDITORS' FOREWORD

DURING 1963, the Council of the Eugenics Society decided to extend the Society's activities by organizing a series of symposia designed to bridge the gap between the biomedical and the social sciences. The first, held in September 1964, under the title *Biological Aspects of Social Problems* was highly successful and fully justified both the publication of the proceedings and the continuation of the projected series. Accordingly, the second symposium, entitled *Genetic and Environmental Factors in Human Ability*, was held on 30th September and 1st October 1965. As on the first occasion, this second meeting brought together people who might otherwise never have had the opportunity to exchange ideas, and it was generally agreed to have been most useful. The proceedings of this meeting, which was opened by Sir Robert Platt, as President of the Eugenics Society, are recorded in the present volume, which we feel will be a worthy successor to the preceding one. For this, the Society is greatly indebted to all those who took an active part in the meeting by contributing formally or in discussion.

As Honorary Treasurer and Honorary Secretary of the Society, we have again accepted formal responsibility for the editing of the present volume, but, as on the previous occasion, the day-to-day work and responsibility has fallen on Mrs K. Hodson, editor of *The Eugenics Review* ; to her are due the best thanks of the Society and of all readers of this book.

J. E. MEADE
A. S. PARKES

CONTENTS

GENERAL INTRODUCTION

SIR ROBERT PLATT

Cambridge

IN writing the General Introduction to this Symposium volume I assume a dual role: first of all as Chairman of the first session of this Symposium and secondly as the new President of the Eugenics Society, an office which I am extremely proud to hold and no little surprised to have been invited to hold. I hope this Society will continue to prosper under my presidency and if it fails to do so I can only say it will not be due to any lack of interest on my part in the kind of lectures and discussions which it is its business to organize.

As a physician I first became interested in genetics when, as a medical student, I read Bateson on Mendelism (though genetics was not taught to medical students very much in those days) and I have spent my life in the study of man. My hobby, you might say, as well as my occupation, has been the fascinating interest of the interplay of genetic and environmental factors in patients and their illnesses, and perhaps even more in their attitudes to those illnesses.

The scope of what is now included under the somewhat elastic title of ' eugenics ' has no doubt changed from time to time since Galton first introduced the term. Rather than attempt at this moment any new definition—and there are already plenty—of what eugenics really comprises, I would draw attention to the wide scope of interest of the Eugenics Society, as shown by the impressive list of past presidents, ending with that very distinguished zoologist, Sir James Gray, and as is shown also by the subject matter of these two Symposia, the first on *Biological Aspects of Social Problems*, and this, the second, on *Genetic and Environmental Factors in Human Ability*.

Our aim is to bring together people from different branches of learning—genetics, sociology, physiology, psychology, education and so on—with a common interest in applying their particular study to the problems of man and especially to the future of man. In order to do this they must—and this is good for them and essential for the rest of us—speak a common language ; it does not have to be the language that is used in mathematical genetics or physics or something of that kind ; it has to be the ordinary English language such as intelligent people like ourselves can listen to and understand. If Arthur Koestler is right in asserting that a new idea, a new conception, a new discovery, is due usually to the coming together of two quite different approaches to a problem, then this Society should be able to throw up new ideas from time to time—the kind of thing (although there will not be many such obvious examples in human history) that Mendel did when he brought together botany and mathematics practically for the first time. However we still have not quite dealt with what is comprised in eugenics because the ' eu ' of eugenics indicates that we consider it part of our job to consider, and then try to judge, *values*. That is always a difficult and dangerous thing to do. It is my view that in the society in which we now live, dominated as it is by scientific and technical achievements, a society which has given up and discarded many old theories and many old beliefs, some intellectuals have gone rather too far in their fear of entering the difficult field of ethics. I do not think it is the function of the Eugenics Society to take on a mantle of omniscience and make pronouncements for all time on these difficult problems, but I do think it should not shirk the ethical issues which immediately arise when the future of man is under consideration.

To come now to the matter of this Symposium, it might seem that the interpretation of human ability would be weighted in favour of intelligence ; I would remind you that this is not the only human ability, neither is it the sole factor in human ability. Intelligence is of basic importance, of course ; but something else, which is difficult to define and which we usually refer to as ' personality ', is also extremely important ; and so also is sheer technical skill, which people often forget in their thinking on human ability. I have from time to time pointed out to my students that there are two almost completely different kinds of learning. Given lectures and discussions, illustrations and so on, plus a reasonable educational background, a student can be made to understand principles of the function of the lungs or of logarithms or something of that kind ; but, given a few lectures and illustrations on the violin, he would still not be able to play a note, nor would he probably play well for many years. These are quite different kinds of learning, but technical skill is an extremely important human ability, interestingly enough, one in which the human race continues to progress: for instance, there is never a big meeting of athletes, such as the Olympic Games, at which records are not broken in one field or another. To return to stringed instruments, when Tchaikovsky wrote his violin concerto, it was turned down by two of the greatest violinists of the time as unplayable. Now, I suppose, it is in the repertoire of every violinist who looks upon himself as being at concerto level.

Some of what I have said would perhaps have been said more appropriately at the end of this Symposium than at the beginning, and I am reminded of something that Sir Geoffrey Jefferson once told me. He was asked to take the chair at a conference and the secretary of the society said to him, " We're rather pushed for time. If you have any introductory remarks, would you mind making them at the end ? " Perhaps that is what I should have done.

THE NATURE AND MEANING OF INTELLIGENCE TESTS

Chairman: Sir Robert Platt

DEVELOPMENT OF CURRENT IDEAS ABOUT INTELLIGENCE TESTS

PHILIP E. VERNON
University of London Institute of Education

IF some of the leading British and American writers on intelligence, such as Burt,[3] R. B. Cattell,[4] Guilford,[8] McNemar [13] and Hunt [12] were asked for their views on intelligence tests, there would be a wide range of disagreement. All I can hope to do is point to certain developments that have been apparent over the past thirty years or so, and then restate what seems to me the position of the majority of middle-of-the-road psychologists.

1. There has been an increasing disinclination to accept the notion of intelligence as an inherited and measureable quality of the individual which simply matures as he grows older, regardless of upbringing and education.

2. The earlier belief in an antithesis between innate intelligence and acquired attainments has largely broken down; in particular the notion of the Achievement Quotient has been discredited. We realize that all types of ability develop through interaction between the maturing organism and a stimulating environment, and are intimately bound up with dynamic personality trends, motivations and social processes. This implies a greater disbelief in the long-term predictive value of the IQ.

3. There has been increasing interest in the psychological processes underlying intellectual performance, the nature of the child's percepts and concepts at different ages which Piaget [16] has stressed, and the study of brain-functioning in the light of information theory and computer models.[14]

4. There has been an increasing tendency to break down a single global intelligence or *g* into a large number of partly distinct ability factors, but attempts to develop differential tests for abilities along different lines, have not in fact met with much success.[23]

5. There is increasing dissatisfaction with the types of multiple-choice items that make up the conventional group intelligence test, and greater realization that performance at these is considerably affected by previous practice and coaching. The increasing use of machine-scored tests, to facilitate the testing of large numbers, has not helped matters. At the same time there has been little progress in developing less restricted item forms, though the current concern with so-called divergent thinking and creative abilities is of interest.

6. There have, then, been many and varied critical attacks on the earlier, rather naïve, view of intelligence-testing commonly held in the 1920s—a view which is still all too widespread among teachers and educated laymen generally. But in spite of these attacks there has been no decline in the practice of applying tests—whether Binet or Wechsler tests for clinical purposes or of group tests for educational and vocational selection and guidance, or in research investigations. Currently the Department of Education and Science is giving heavy financial backing to the British Psychological Society's five-year project for the production of a new British Intelligence Scale for individual testing of 5 – 12-year-old children, under the direction of Professor Warburton of Manchester University. And it is estimated by Henry Chauncey, President of the American Educational Testing Service, that 150 million standardized tests were applied in American schools and colleges in 1964, a large proportion of which were tests of academic aptitude—I will not call them ' intelligence tests '.

Turning now to the major controversies which still centre round the problem of heredity and environment: we realize that this problem is much more complicated than was at first thought, and that there is no simple answer in terms of ' so much variance attributable to genetic, so much to environmental, components '. Intelligence is not, of course, a definite unitary entity, like colour blindness—dependent on particular genes. It is merely a name for the overall efficiency and level of complexity of an individual's cognitive processes. Godfrey Thomson [18] referred to the underlying mental structures as ' bonds ', Thorndike as ' connections ' or ' associations '. Each of these terms bears an unduly mechanistic flavour, and modern psychology prefers the notion of 'schemata' as described by F. C. Bartlett [1] and J. Piaget, or what Miller, Galanter and Pribram [14] calls 'plans'. In the course of development the individual builds up an enormous storehouse of concepts and skills, by means of which he interprets and copes with the world more or less effectively. As D. O. Hebb [10] and Piaget [16] have shown, these skills or plans are developed through use, in reacting to environmental stimulation. Except, perhaps, some of the earliest and simplest sensory-motor reflexes, we cannot regard them as 'given' in the innate structure of the nervous system, nor as maturing *in vacuo* purely through genetic determination. We *learn* to perceive, to imagine, to reason, to judge; and, as Harlow [9] pointed out, we learn how to learn just as much as we learn how to ride a bicycle or learn spelling and arithmetic. It is true, of course, that without the necessary genes we could not develop physically or mentally at all, and also that some individuals have more favourable genes for the acquisition of cognitive schemata than others do. We can go a bit further and state that some individuals are more favoured with genes that underlie musical, numerical and other specialized types of learning. But we still have to regard general intelligence, or more specialized number and other abilities, as developed through interaction with environment, and must therefore reject the notion that any tests can reveal the innate components of mental aptitudes. As Hebb puts it, there is an Intelligence A, the genetic potentiality which is non-observable and non-measurable. The Intelligence B which we observe in a person's behaviour and thinking is the product of the interaction between Intelligence A and environment. This distinction between the genotype and the phenotype is entirely in accordance with general genetic theory: a healthy plant requires good seed, but it also requires suitable warmth, moisture and nutriment. Similarly the human being requires physical and emotional security and a richly stimulating environment if his intelligence is to develop.

One more distinction is useful at this point—that between observed Intelligence B and measured intelligence, which I have referred to elsewhere [21] as 'intelligence C'. Intelligence

C is simply a sampling of B which can be scored in IQ or other units. The tests that we apply may or may not yield a fairly adequate sampling of all the concepts and skills that go to make up B.

How can we be so confident that there are inherited differences in potentiality, i.e. Intelligence A? Why not accept J. B. Watson's claim that, if given complete control of environment, he could bring up different children to be anything he liked—doctor, artist, beggarman or thief? It is usually supposed that the moderate resemblance in Intelligence C of offspring to parents and the very close resemblance of identical twins to one another give evidence of genetic determination, but both these resemblances could, of course, be explained by environmental influence. Identical twins tend to be brought up much more alike than ordinary siblings or fraternal twins and thus would be expected to show higher correlations. The evidence from identical twins brought up apart is somewhat more convincing though, to my mind, impossible to interpret, since the members of separated pairs are unlikely to be placed in different environments at random. Thus Burt's [3] separated pairs show closer resemblances than those of Newman, Freeman and Holzinger,[15] probably because the environments of most of the former were fairly similar. Much more impressive is Newman's finding that, the greater the dissimilarity of environments, the lower the degree of resemblance in IQ. No; the really convincing evidence of genetic determination is: first, the correlation between the intelligence of orphans or foster children and that of their true parents who have had nothing to do with their upbringing; and second, the fact that children in the same family often differ so widely in intelligence from their parents or from one another. If socio-economic, cultural and health conditions were all-important in producing Intelligence B and C, we would surely expect a much higher correlation than 0·5 between parents and offspring or between siblings. Only genetic theory seems capable of explaining why professional parents sometimes have a dull child, or uneducated lower working class parents a very bright one.

Now, though we must admit the importance of genetic influences in observed and measured intelligence, this does not mean that any tests, however good a sampling they give of Intelligence B, can ever provide us with even a moderately reliable estimate of the Intelligence A of an individual or of a group. Experts in this field, such as Burt in England and Burks [2] in America, have estimated the genetic component in intelligence test scores as 75–80 per cent ; and Burt claims that, by using suitable individual tests, including non-language tests, and making a clinical assessment of the likely effects of abnormal environmental conditions, he can arrive at a measure of a child's intelligence which represents to even 90 per cent the genetic component. I do not regard such figures as realistic, because the relative importance of the environmental factors clearly varies with the range of environmental differences. I would agree that, when all members of a cultural group are brought up under fairly similar circumstances and receive a fairly standard education, the major part of their variance in intelligence is hereditary. But when there are wide differences in socio-economic level and education, such as those between Western European (or North American) children and children in underdeveloped societies, the environmental factors are much more potent. Moreover they can affect allegedly culture-free tests at least as much as conventional verbal tests. I have recently had the opportunity to apply the same 4 – 5-hour battery of group and individual tests to groups of boys around eleven years old in S.E. England and the remote Hebridean islands, to West Indians in Jamaica, to Canadian Indians in Alberta and to Eskimos north of the Arctic Circle. Their comparative performance in vocabulary and educational tests certainly reflected the degree to which standard English was used in their homes, and the extent of their education. But among the various groups of boys with similar linguistic handicaps, the scores on performance tests like Kohs Blocks and a non-verbal Matrices-type test ranged all the way from a mean quotient of 75 for West Indians to 93 for Bush Eskimos (where the English mean is 100 and the Standard Deviation 15). It appeared that the nature of their upbringing, whether it was restrictive or permissive, whether it discouraged or encouraged resourcefulness, masculine identification and exploiting one's physical environment, was mainly responsible for these differences in the grasping of patterns and reasoning skills.

Now let us turn to the other main source of controversy concerning intelligence and intelligence tests: is there a general, unitary ability—Spearman's *g*, or must we recognize a large number of distinctive, even if overlapping, faculties or factors, as do Thurstone,[19] Guilford,[8] and the majority of American psychometrists? This does not seem to me a difficult problem, provided one admits that factors are merely clusters of similar skills and does not reify them into fundamental components or chemical elements, as it were, of mind. Consider the analogy of school marks.* It is perfectly legitimate to find each pupil's average marks in all subjects and to give him an overall mark for his general level of achievement. Alternatively, the headmaster may prefer to have a total mark for performance in Arts subjects, another for science-plus-maths, and, in the typical grammar school, the correlation between these two major groups would be fairly low. Thirdly, it is perfectly meaningful to list the marks for each separate subject in the curriculum, though naturally these will show generally positive correlations. Fourthly, one can break down still further and score the pupils separately for spelling, handwriting, etc. within the language group; and for arithmetic, algebra and geometry; and so on. These minor group factors tend to have much in common but also show a fair amount of distinctiveness.

The same principle applies to the organization of mental abilities in general; for we can group in many different ways, some more broad, some more detailed. However, a good deal of controversy and confusion has arisen, partly because different factorists use a variety of techniques of analysis and rotation and have varying standards of statistical significance, but largely because most American factorial studies are carried out on college students or other highly selected groups, most

* Factor analysts will realize that this analogy is not quite correct in so far as group factors, e.g. in science, spelling, etc. represent the variance in these marks after allowing for the variance attributable to *g* or other higher-order factors. American oblique primary factors would, however, be more comparable to separate sets of school marks.

British studies on relatively heterogeneous populations such as complete age-groups of pupils, or army recruits.[23] Since test correlations are necessarily lowered in homogeneous groups, Americans favour a large number of independent primary factors, with no general factor. Guilford claims to have established some sixty factors of intellect, and hundreds of others have been described by other psychometrists. Recently, however, there have been signs of a reaction. Quinn McNemar [13] refers to ' the fragmentation of ability into more and more factors of less and less importance ', and both he and Lloyd Humphreys [11] advocate a return to something like the British model of a strong general intelligence factor and subsidiary group factors representing more specialized skills.

At the same time Thurstone, Guilford and others are justified in claiming that a single, vague and indeterminate IQ hardly does justice to the richness and variety of mental life, especially at higher intellectual levels. Intelligence B has many different aspects, according to the kinds of situations or tasks, though these still tend to have much in common when measured in unselected populations. For example, it is easy to establish partially distinctive factors in spatial or numerical, as contrasted with verbal, test materials, in rote memorizing tasks, in speeded clerical type tasks, and so on. It has proved much more difficult to differentiate psychological faculties such as attention, inductive and deductive reasoning, logical memorizing, imagination, creativity, etc., the main reason being that we cannot readily devise tests which provide adequate sampling of any one faculty alone. Test performance usually involves a great many other processes which we cannot disentangle or control, such as previous familiarity with that kind of material, or quickness in acquiring facility with it, sophistication or practice with tests in general, comprehension of the rather elaborate printed instructions that the tester supplies, wise use of the time allowance and of the possibilities of guessing if the test is speeded, and persistence and interest in the task if it is untimed, and so on. A test may appear to involve some particular faculty, but we seldom know much about the processes testees actually use, and two people may well attain the same score using very different processes. In other words,

Intelligence C and the various statistical factors into which it can be broken down may be a poor reflection of the intellectual abilities B that the person normally uses in real-life situations.

Let us now see how these ideas apply in the field of creativity. Guilford,[8] Getzels and Jackson,[7] Torrance [20] and others have pointed out that almost all conventional group tests demand convergent or conformist thinking ; the testee has to choose the answer which the test constructor has decided to be the right one. Tests can be devised, however, in which there is no one right answer but where the score is based on fluency or number of ideas, on how diverse they are, how unusual, or even how clever and original—though the latter obviously involves somewhat subjective evaluation. These tests of divergent thinking, they claim, measure a very different factor or factors from the verbal IQ, and they have argued strongly that the American educational system, with its tests and objective examinations, together with parent, teacher and peer-group pressures towards conformity, are stifling the creative abilities of the growing generation. Dr Hudson discusses these arguments elsewhere in this Symposium ; here I am concerned to point out that the psychometric basis of so-called creativity tests is decidedly shaky. The kind of tests that Guilford, Torrance and others are using are poor samples of original thought or creative invention in the generally accepted sense, and so far there is little evidence that we could select more desirable students by using them instead of, or in addition to, convergent tests. In other words, we are not entitled to identify Divergent Ability C with Creativity B. Moreover, it is doubtful how far tests of divergent thinking really yield a distinctive factor or factors. True, the correlations with convergent tests tend to be low in selected or homogeneous populations, partly because the reliabilities of the tests themselves are low. In less restricted populations they show considerable overlapping with standard tests, and the extent of correlation between different creativity measures themselves does not seem to be much higher. If, instead of using group tests as our criterion of intelligence, we used the individual Stanford-Binet tests, where the testee supplies his responses in his own words, it might be still more difficult to establish any distinctive divergent factors.

We now come back to the general question of what intelligence tests measure. The realistic answer is that they measure the average efficiency with which testees cope with the kinds of problems the tester chooses to include. Different choices of subtests will give similar but by no means identical *g*'s. Thus, most group tests are strongly weighted in favour of verbal comprehension and reasoning, partly because items of this kind are traditional, easy to construct and convenient to administer and score, partly because they give rather highly valid predictions of educational capacity over the ensuing two to five years. Other test authors prefer to reduce the verbal bias for one reason or another, and such batteries will still correlate moderately highly with verbal ones. But they give a less useful sampling of the thinking skills employed either at school or in daily life, because we mainly think in words and because the pictorial or diagrammatic material of the tests is artificial. Possibly, however, such tests are more valid than verbal tests in relation to mathematical and scientific education. Verbal group tests are genuinely useful, because they provide quite a good sampling of academic thinking over the mental age of about ten to fifteen years. They seem to have poorer validity at higher levels, in grammar or public schools or universities. Hudson suggests that this is because the problems they include are too trivial ; that the really able student can express his full ability only on larger and more complex tasks in which he is truly interested. They tend to work better in America than in England, partly because most American High School and college populations are less highly selected, so that correlations are higher, but also because the criterion of good achievement in the American educational system so often consists of multiple-choice or objective examinations, which have much more in common with the psychologist's academic aptitude tests than do the criteria that British educationists chiefly look for.

Individual tests like the Stanford-Binet represent yet another sampling of intellectual skills. They correlate imperfectly with group tests because they are less biased by such irrelevancies as facility in doing multiple-choice items at speed, comprehending printed directions, etc. For the same reason they probably provide the most representative cross-section yet attained of daily life cognitive schemata over the 2 to 15-year mental age range. In addition, either group or individual tests may be composed of spatial, numerical, clerical, musical, creativity or other sorts of items ; and these still overlap the ordinary intelligence test to a considerable extent, though their content may make them more relevant to technical, clerical, musical or other criteria.

There is no sharp distinction between any of these and so-called achievement or attainment tests in, say, reading, arithmetic, science, etc. ; for I have already tried to make clear that Intelligence B should be regarded as a kind or class of attainments. However, the former do involve more general skills of comprehending, reasoning, judging, etc. which are transferable to a wide variety of situations, whereas the latter usually involve more specialized schemata, and depend more on the amount and quality of school instruction and the pupil's interest in the topic. Again, the development of general intellectual skills, while certainly stimulated by good or depressed by poor, schooling also reflects exercise outside the school—at home, in leisure activities and so forth. Thus, in a rather narrow sense, one can use intelligence tests as predictors of educational potential, not because they are pure measures of Intelligence A, but because a child who has developed effective schemata in his daily-life thinking and behaviour, through some combination of good genes with fortunate circumstances, might normally be expected to be able to use these schemata in the school situation also. Although the practice, common among educational psychologists, of concentrating their remedial work almost exclusively on children whose educational age is lower than their mental age is riddled with fallacies (as Pidgeon [17] and others, including myself,[22] have shown elsewhere), yet recent experiments by a student of mine, Mr Hugh Lytton, indicate that the IQs of backward children do correlate to a small but useful extent with gains in reading and arithmetic following remedial treatment. The intelligence test is a useful predictor also around the age of

10–15 years, when children are changing school, embarking on new subjects, or entering jobs or technical training. Their performance in, say, mathematics may be considerably affected by ease or difficulty of adaptation to the new social environment, the new teacher and the more advanced curriculum ; hence previous performance in arithmetic may be a weaker predictor than their generalized intellectual skills.

Could not one still argue that intelligence test results are a better indicator of genetic capacity than attainment tests ? I would agree, with considerable caution, mainly on the grounds that parent-child and sibling correlations tend to be lower for the former than the latter. Several investigators, among them Elizabeth Fraser,[6] have shown that attainment scores or teachers' assessments are rather more strongly associated with social class and parental attitudes to education than are intelligence test scores. Hence the abolition of intelligence tests in any eleven plus selection procedure tends to increase the social class bias, even if not very markedly, and to result in fewer grammar school places going to bright children from poor homes. Again, while accepting Douglas's [5] recent findings that IQ change from age 8 to age 11 is affected in much the same manner as attainment change is affected by home and school influences, I would not go so far as he does in ignoring any differences between these two types of measures.

REFERENCES

1. Bartlett, F. C. 1958. *Thinking.* London. Allen and Unwin.
2. Burks, B. S. 1928. The relative influence of nature upon mental development. 27th *Yrbk. Nat. Soc. Stud. Educ.* **1**, 219.
3. Burt, C. L. 1955. The evidence for the concept of intelligence. *Brit. J. educ. Psychol.* **25**, 158.
4. Cattell, R. B. 1963. Theory of fluid and crystallized intelligence: a critical experiment. *J. educ. Psychol.* **54**, 1.
5. Douglas, J. W. B. 1964. *The Home and the School.* London. MacGibbon and Kee.
6. Fraser, E. 1959. *Home Environment and the School.* London. University of London Press.
7. Getzels, J. W. and Jackson, P. W. 1962. *Creativity and Intelligence.* New York. Wiley.

8. Guilford, J. P. 1959. Three faces of intellect. *Amer. Psychologist* **14**, 469.
9. Harlow, H. F. 1949. The formation of learning sets. *Psychol. Rev.* **56**, 51.
10. Hebb, D. O. 1948. *The Organization of Behavior*. New York. Wiley.
11. Humphreys, L. G. 1962. The organization of human abilities. *Amer. Psychologist* **17**, 475.
12. Hunt, J. McV. 1961. *Intelligence and Experience*. New York. Ronald Press.
13. McNemar, Q. 1964. Lost: our intelligence? Why? *Amer. Psychologist* **19**, 871.
14. Miller, G. A., Galanter, E. and Pribram, K. H. 1960. *Plans and the Structure of Behavior*. New York. Holt.
15. Newman, H. H., Freeman, F. N. and Holzinger, K. J. 1937. *Twins: A Study of Heredity and Environment*. Chicago. University of Chicago Press.
16. Piaget, J. 1950. *The Psychology of Intelligence*. London. Routledge and Kegan Paul.
17. Pidgeon, D. A., Yates, A. and Brimer, M. A. 1957. Ability and attainment. *Bull. Nat. Found. educ. Res.* **10**, 22.
18. Thomson, G. H. 1939. *The Factorial Analysis of Human Ability*. London. University of London Press.
19. Thurstone, L. L. 1938. Primary mental abilities. *Psychometric Monogr.* No. 1. Chicago. University of Chicago Press.
20. Torrance, E. P. 1962. Measurement and development of the creative thinking abilities. *Yrbk. of Educ.: The Gifted Child* 125.
21. Vernon, P. E. 1955. The assessment of children. Univ. of London Instit. Educ., *Studies in Education* Vol. 7, 189.
22. Vernon, P. E. 1958. The relation of intelligence to educational backwardness. *Educ. Rev.* **11**, 7.
23. Vernon, P. E. 1965. Ability factors and environmental influences. *Amer. Psychologist* **20**. In Press.

SOME ASPECTS OF THE RELATIONSHIP BETWEEN COMMUNICATION AND PERFORMANCES IN TESTS *

B. B. BERNSTEIN and D. YOUNG

Sociological Research Unit,
University of London Institute of Education

IN this paper we shall give an interim report of some of the findings of the Sociological Research Unit which have a bearing on the major topic for this session. We shall first give a general outline of the research undertaken and then discuss briefly the sample, the methods used, the procedures for analysing the data and finally some interim findings. There is, unfortunately, no time to discuss the theoretical perspective which is influencing the research.

Essentially the Research Unit is making a comparison between forms of interaction between mother and children within middle- and working-class families and their responsiveness towards education. We are concerned to relate these forms of family interaction and their educational procedures to linguistic development and control by infant school children. We are also concerned with the possible relationships between forms of linguistic development and the child's cognitive and social procedures. Our aim is, ultimately, to construct a communication profile for a family, to group families sharing similar profiles, and then to examine forms of a child's speech in terms of such profiles. In this way we shall dispense with social class as a major independent variable, substituting instead a communication profile. We would then be able to relate such a profile to a child's performance on ability tests, his general education attainment, his form of speech, his social and cognitive procedures. We have some reason to believe that the forms of family interaction which shape patterns of

* This research is supported by grants from the Department of Education and Science and the Ford Foundation.

communication have a social origin. At the moment, however, we are a long way from producing a communication profile.

The major sample consists of approximately 300 families living in a predominantly working-class area and 150 families from a predominantly middle-class area. We are following the children of these families for a period of three years from the point of entry into the infant school. The methods used are: first, a social survey ; second, an intensive non-questionnaire approach to a selected group of families ; and third, experimental studies of the children's speech.

All the mothers of the children were visited and a tape-recorded interview was obtained in the July preceding the child's entry to school. This interview consisted of mothers talking freely in response to a number of questions. Mothers also completed a number of closed schedules by ticking, marking, or listing a range of items. In the free section of this interview we were concerned with how the mother prepared the child for school, how she drew the boundary between family and school, her concept of brightness and of play, how she controlled the child, how she explained things to the child, what procedures she possessed for dealing with problems which might arise when the child was at school. This interview also gave us a selective sample of the mother's speech in different areas. The closed or tick schedules, or at least the ones with which we shall be concerned here, dealt with such things as the way the mother coped with questions from the child, with her willingness to enter into verbal interaction with her child, her views on the uses of toys, and the nature of the boundary she drew between herself and the school.

After three weeks in school the children were given three ability tests, and a language sample was also taken. At the end of the first year at school the free, informal and unobserved speech for a whole day at school was collected from fifty children The teachers in the fourteen schools at the end of this year judged the responsiveness of the children to school in terms of types of verbal interactions and also estimated the degree of brightness of the children.

We shall now describe the results of some of the closed schedules completed by the mothers and the teachers in relation to the children's ability test scores at age five for the families living in the predominantly working-class area. We are concerned, first, to show the relationships between purely demographic variables, such as social class and family size, and ability test scores ; then to show the relationships between family interaction variables and ability test scores and the teacher's perception of the child at school ; finally to show relationships when demographic variables are held constant and noting the influence of the family interaction variables.

We have in all cases been interested in the behaviour of certain critical groups and a X^2 analysis has been used so far in our calculations ; this will give way shortly to a multiple correlational analysis. We had hoped that it would be completed in time for this paper.

We start by explaining the bases of the indices we have constructed for the analysis of the data, taking first the social class index. It is important to remember that this sample is relatively homogeneous and that ' high social class ' (as we shall refer to it) does not reach the conventional middle class of the major and minor professions, business men, administrators and higher supervisory groups. The index we constructed is very similar to that used by Douglas. It consists of a scale based upon the mother's and father's terminal education and occupation. On this basis we were able to assign families to three socio-economic groups, High, Medium, Low, broadly but not wholly, corresponding to semi-skilled and unskilled ; skilled ; white collar lower supervisory positions.

Now let us examine the family-size index. As our sample consists of families at various stages of completion, it was necessary to correct family size by the age of the mother. The correction we used was over and under thirty years of age. The split in family size to be used in this discussion is between families of two or one, and three or more. We are, of course, able to sort in terms of smaller or larger family, younger or older mother, etc.

The interaction index was made up of the mother's responses to three closed schedules. One schedule related to the way the mother dealt with questions from the child: from her replies we computed an avoidance score in terms of how much she avoided, escaped from, or refused to answer the question. The second schedule dealt with the mother's willingness to enter into verbal interaction with the child in a range of social situations. From the replies on both of these schedules we constructed the communication component of the interaction index on a five-point scale. For our present purpose it has been dichotomized into High or Low so that it can be treated as an attribute present or absent. In the same way we can treat the family size and the social class index as favourable or unfavourable attributes.

The third schedule dealt with the mother's views on the use of toys. The mother had to mark six possible functions of the uses of toys in order of importance. In scoring we used only those which she considered the most important and least important. If she chose ' to find out about things ' as the most important, this was treated as a positive attribute. If she chose as the *least* important the item we considered as indicating the smallest desire to interact with the child, this was also treated as a positive attribute. This item was ' to free mother so that she could do other things '.

A mother with a lowest interaction index would be one who scored low on the communication component and put first and last on the uses-of-toys-schedule anything other than the two items I have mentioned. A mother with the highest interaction index would be one who scored high on the communication component and placed ' to find out about things ' first on the toy schedule and ' to free the mother etc.' last on it. Intervening positions between these two extremes can be, and are, dealt with.

Now we come to the ability tests given to the children. For a number of reasons we did not give the Stanford-Binet ; but this year all the children will be given the WISC. We took advice and gave the five-year-olds the Crichton Scale, which is a word-definition test ; the English version of the Peabody Picture Vocabulary Test, which is essentially a test of vocabulary of recognition ; and the Children's version of the Raven's Progressive Matrices, a test of relatively non-verbal ability. In reporting some of our results we shall talk of Combined Test Score, whether High, Medium or Low. For a child to be in a High group, he would have had to score High on at least two of the tests, and to be in a Low group to have scored low on at least two of the tests ; similarly for Medium. But this category also included a small number who scored High, Medium and Low on the three tests.

It must be added that children were assigned to an individual test category in terms of the distribution of scores we obtained from our sample. Now each of these indices—social class, corrected family size and the interaction index—was expected to be related to the test scores of the children grouped in the three categories: high, medium and low scores. More than this—within each index, variations in the score Low, High were also considered to bear a similar relation to an ability score. Thus, we might expect to find that a very high proportion of children coming from small families, with older mothers scoring high on the interaction index, belonging to our so-called high socio-economic group, would have high ability scores. With less favourable shifts in each index we might expect a corresponding drop in ability score. The results we found are given in the following paragraphs.

First let us consider the demographic variables—social class and family size. Social class was not significantly related to any of the ability test scores. Indeed, it reached only an 0·05 level of significance with the Crichton Scale (verbal definition test) when compared with the lowest and the highest social class groups. It must, however, be remembered that the social class range within our sample is certainly a very restricted one. Family size is, however, very powerfully related to each ability test score and to the Combined Test Score at a 0·001 level of confidence.

Next let us turn to the relation among social class and family size and the interaction index and then to the relation between the interaction index and ability scores. There is no relation between our family-size index and our restricted social class groups. But there is a very powerful relation between social class and the interaction index at a 0·001 level of confidence. The relation between family size and the interaction index is significant but very much weaker at 0·02 level of confidence.

We now turn to the relation between the interaction index

and the ability test scores classified as high, medium and low. The interaction index is very powerfully related to the Combined Test Score, as strongly as family size at a 0·001 level of confidence, and relates to each individual test at a 0·01 level of confidence. Thus the interaction index produces as strong a relation with combined ability scores as does family size, whereas the relation between family size and the interaction index is relatively weak, although significant.

Our next step will be to examine the effect of differences in the interaction index on ability test scores holding family size constant. If a family is small, two or less, differences in the interaction index have no significant effect on ability test score. However, if the family is large, three or more, a difference in the interaction index is significantly related at a 0·01 level of confidence to the Combined Test Score, and individually to the Crichton and to the EPVT. So a high interaction index for a large family gives promise of a significantly greater proportion of children with high ability scores compared with large families with a low interaction score. This finding would seem to be of particular significance when we consider the normal social class gradient for family size. The interaction index discriminates between large families and, with an adjustment which cannot be detailed here, it is also capable of similar discrimination between small families.

Before turning to the consideration of some findings which concern the mother's relation with the school and the teacher's estimate of the child's brightness, we shall look briefly at some relations with the score on the Matrices, the relatively non-verbal test. We have shown that there is a powerful relation between family size and non-verbal test score. There is, however, a significant relationship between the mother's choice of the uses of toys and the child's chances of being in the high category on the Matrices test. A point worth making here is that the communication component of the interaction index is not at all related to the child's Matrices score.

Next, we consider some aspects of the child's behaviour in school and the mother's relation to the school, in terms of the variables we have discussed. In this sample the children attend fourteen schools, and their teachers were asked to answer a number of questions about the children at the end of the first year. One of these questions called for an estimate of ability—was the child bright, average or weak? Now—and this is of some importance—the social class of the child was found to bear no relation to these estimates. Family size and the interaction index each separately related at a 0·001 level of confidence to the teacher's judgement. But, when family size was held constant, the score on the interaction index was significantly related to the teacher's estimate, and the index discriminated within small and within large families. Thus, the proportion of children judged by the teachers to be bright is related to whether a family has a favourable or unfavourable interaction index within both large families and small families.

Lastly, we mention a finding which has a bearing on the mother's relation to the school. In the course of an interview, the mother was given a schedule containing a range of behaviour patterns of her child, and she had to judge whether they were entirely her own responsibility, or a responsibility shared between the school and herself, or entirely the school's concern. A scale was constructed, based upon the number of items a mother considered to be matters of shared or joint responsibility. We examined each mother's score on this scale of joint responsibility together with four variables we have discussed, namely social class, family size, children's test score, and the interaction index. Of these four variables, the interaction index alone significantly correlated with the score—if high—made by mothers on our scale of shared responsibility. Minimally, this scale shows that these mothers regard the school as being as deeply concerned with the child's development as they are themselves.

Thus, the interaction index not only relates to the children's ability test scores and discriminates between families of equal size, but also is related to the teacher's judgement of the degree of brightness of the child, and to the mother's opting for a position of joint concern or responsibility with the school across a range of different aspects of the child's behaviour.

One possible explanation of the power of this variable in our sample is that the IQ of the child, or that of the mother, or both interacting together, accounts for the quality of the interaction. This matter will be finally decided when we obtain the IQs of the parents, as we intend to do.

Arguments against this view could be put forward, among them the following:

1. The social class range in this sample is very restricted. Among the mothers the difference between the highest and the lowest may not be more than eight IQ points. The IQ range for the children also is somewhat restricted. Nevertheless, the discriminations we have obtained are very powerful.

2. The range of IQs within a family, especially a large family, is likely to be wide. Our data show that there is no relation between the mother's interaction index and the ordinal position of a child when single children in different families are compared, or eldest children with younger members of the same family.

3. Were the interaction index a measure of the mother's IQ alone, since this is presumably related to the child's IQ, then the ability test scores of the child would be expected to show some relation to the joint-responsibility scale. In fact, there is no such relation.

4. The relation between interaction index and ability tests is very unlikely to hold in the case of the middle- and upper-middle-class sample.

5. Finally, there are good cross-cultural reasons for believing that forms of familial interaction have in large measure a social origin.

CONCLUSION

It is quite clear that the limits of endeavour are set organically, but that the rate of mental development and the functioning level are influenced by the quality of the environment. There is often a gap between potential capacity and actually developed ability. The interaction index and its development may be a short step, along with many others, in making explicit the processes which produce what in our culture we call intelligent behaviour and educational attainment. Moreover, many children, who grow up in family settings where the communication process is inadequate, as judged by the school, may be fundamentally handicapped for social reasons over which they have no control. The evidence offered here, in conjunction with other evidence, may point to a need for an enlargement of work in the area of communication in infant schools where children come from homes with problems of inadequate communication and interaction. Indeed, we may have to think much more seriously about nursery school provision as well as the more material provision of decent houses and decent schools.

Communication patterns are rooted deep within a given culture ; indeed they are the expression of it, and great care and sensitivity are required of those who wish to modify them. For some children school is an experience of development of their linguistic and relational procedures ; for others it will undoubtedly be an experience of change in these same procedures. We can temper this process both for the family and for the child, only if we have a more systematic knowledge of family interactions and their resultant patterns of communication.

SOCIAL BACKGROUND, INTELLIGENCE AND SCHOOL STRUCTURE: AN INTERACTION ANALYSIS

HILDE T. HIMMELWEIT
London School of Economics

UNTIL recently, social scientists tended to look for one or two explanatory factors of the behaviour they studied. As a result, tenuous relationships between variables have tended to be stretched beyond their statistical or theoretical justifications. This was particularly so where such relationships had social implications. Two examples come to mind: the first concerns the link between broken homes and delinquency. Study after study has established a significant, but extremely low, relationship between the two ; textbook after textbook mentions the relationship, until broken homes have come to be regarded as the main causal factor in producing delinquent behaviour. It is as if frequency were substituted for importance. This is not so. The correlations remain low ; the exceptions continue to be numerous.

The second example comes from the field of education and concerns the relation between social background and educational attainment. Correlations between social class and O- and A-level performance and between social class and early leaving tend to be in the region of 0·25.[6, 7] These results certainly show that many thousands of children do not realize their intellectual potential and that this constitutes a serious social problem requiring remedial action. However, the relationship is still a weak one ; the question we need to ask, and one which has rarely been examined, is why the effect of home, the principal socializing agent, is not stronger.

There are four reasons for the preference for oversimplified explanations.

The first is the social scientist's desire for order and simplicity, which drives him to the almost hopeless search for *the* significant dimension.

The second lies in the separateness of the disciplines, particularly of sociology and psychology, which is still characteristic of social science in this country. Quite often sociologists and social psychologists study the same phenomenon, but do so from different points of view ; this results, in the one instance, in an oversimplified model of motivation and learning and, in the other, in a neglect of a subtler understanding of the way in which social forces impinge upon the individual's outlook and behaviour. There have been few genuinely interdisciplinary studies.

The third reason is practical ; it concerns money and co-operation. A multidimensional analysis of social or psychological phenomena requires that we gather data about the same individuals or groups from different angles. This is expensive and demands much co-operation from educators and administrators. As long as each specialist is confident in the adequacy of his own preferred explanation, no such requests will be made. Only too often at the beginning of a scientific paper one finds a statement by the author that certain data could not be gathered because the school or institution would not give more time. This is an argument which I find very unconvincing. Teachers and educational authorities are interested and genuine partners in research, provided the reasons for asking for additional time are stated persuasively. My experience in carrying out an inquiry into effects of television on children has convinced me of this. In that study more than 400 class teachers, drawn from 120 schools co-operated ; the teachers gave fully of their own time, and, in addition, permitted us to test the same children on several occasions—nine hours in all.

The last difficulty, lack of facilities for quick, complex statistical analysis, has now fortunately been overcome. Access to computers is a necessary, though not a sufficient, condition for this type of interaction analysis.

In the field of education in recent years, increasing emphasis is being placed on the need for interaction analysis and for linking the characteristics of the school with those of pupil and home when trying to account for differences in scholastic performance. The studies of Douglas,[1] Wiseman [10] and Warburton [9] illustrate this well. These studies of children drawn from a large number of schools, usually on a random basis, examine the children and classify the schools on a number of criteria. They show how, across given social classes and within a particular social class and ability level, the children's school attainments differ, depending on certain characteristics of the school.

The study that I shall be describing carries this type of analysis one step further.* It examines how the different expectations and norms which the child brings to the school influence his response to it. Instead of drawing on a random sample from a large number of schools, this study is concerned with a few schools only and examines the effect of the school on its entire thirteen- to fourteen-year-old intake. Essentially, it amounts to a case study of each school and to an examination of the way in which the organization of the school affects, and is in its turn influenced by, its intake of pupils.

I am singling out selected aspects of a broader follow-up study on which I am currently engaged. The study began some fifteen years ago when I became interested in examining how far the social class differences in child upbringing found in the United States applied to this country and, secondly, how far with our selective secondary school system the effect of sponsored mobility interacted with styles of upbringing characteristic of different social classes.†

Our sample of over 600 thirteen- to fourteen-year-old boys consisted of the entire third forms of nine boys' schools in the Greater London area ; four were grammar and five were secondary modern schools.

By means of open-ended questions, projective tests and inventories, information was sought from the boys about their attitude to schools and to teachers, their relationship with

* The study is being financed by the Science Research Council and by the Department of Education.

† Sponsored mobility is a term coined by Turner [8] which suggests that the working class child who gains entry into the grammar school is propelled into upward mobility since the majority of the jobs to which grammar school pupils go tend to be white collar jobs. By contrast, entry into a secondary modern school may lead to downward mobility for children from middle class homes.

their peers and their parents, their interests and leisure activities, their aspirations and their social attitudes. In addition, we obtained information about the social background of home and, through the teachers, about the boys' performance and behaviour at school, as well as their intelligence ratings at age eleven.[4]

Ten years later we were able to re-interview 74 per cent of the boys ($N = 463$), now aged 23-24, to obtain their educational and vocational history, their attitude to further education and work, their retrospective impressions about school, and their social and political attitudes. The follow-up part of the inquiry was done by means of exhaustive interviews. In addition, each young man completed a questionnaire at home, providing supplementary information (80 per cent returned these). On both occasions personality tests were given.

The follow-up study is being analysed from a number of different viewpoints.[5] I shall be singling out here those aspects which show the complex interaction between the characteristics of the school and those of the child and his background.

To illustrate the type of analysis which we carried out, I shall concentrate first on the problem of early leaving within grammar schools. The analysis was carried out jointly with Mr D. Young and Mr W. Brandis. The Ministry of Education's *Early Leaving Report* [6] and *Statistics*[7], including the most recent, have shown the link between the social background of the child and his age of leaving: the higher the social class, the greater the likelihood that the boy will complete his secondary education. Our data showed the expected trend (Table I).

These figures show that it was the norm for middle-class pupils to stay at school and for the working class pupils to leave early. If this is so, we should not look for *one set* of variables which explain early leaving across social classes, but rather for those variables in each group which account for deviant behaviour among its members. Thus, in the working class group we need an explanation as to why some pupils stayed the course, and in the middle-class group, why some left early. This approach has proved rewarding.

First, we found that a preliminary, but noteworthy,

decision to leave or to stay was made soon after entry into the grammar school. This is contrary to the views expressed in the *Early Leaving Report*,[6] in which it is suggested that the decision is triggered off around age fifteen or sixteen when the boy sees his contemporaries from neighbouring secondary modern schools go out to work and so gain adult status. When we asked the boys at thirteen, i.e. only two years after entering the grammar school, when, if they were free to choose, they would like to leave, 58 per cent of the working-class and 36 per cent of the middle-class pupils wanted to leave at sixteen or

TABLE I

Grammar School Sample ($N = 263$)

Father's Occupation	N	Per cent who left before the Age of 17
Professional/supervisory	63	41
Routine white collar	62	44
Skilled manual	91	63
Semi/unskilled manual	47	64

earlier. Of the potential early leavers, 81 per cent of the working class and 58 per cent of the middle class pupils in fact left early. The wish to leave early and the readiness to translate wish into action varied with social background. The correlation between expressed wish at thirteen and actual leaving age was +0·386 for the middle and +0·437 for the working-class pupils. (Both correlations are significant at the 0·001 level.)

Second, our data relating to the boy's attitudes to school, teachers and peers and his own assessment of his school performance helped to explain some of the underlying motivation. Once again, the set of variables operative in one social group proved less significant in another. The detailed analysis will be described in a forthcoming publication. In summary, the following picture emerged: the working-class boy would stay if he felt accepted and experienced real success; lack of failure was not sufficient. The middle-class boy, on the other hand, would stay whether he experienced success or not and would leave *only* if the failure experienced at school, or stress at school, reinforced by problems at home, proved overwhelming. The role of psychological variables is thus modified by sociological factors.

These findings suggest that for the working-class boy at the time of the study, school was an *ambiguous* situation, a problem to be solved. Gaining a grammar school place was not part of his norm expectation. When he joined the grammar school, he was an interested, yet somewhat detached, participant: how far he subsequently learnt to identify with the norms and values of the school depended, in part, on how much the school showed him that he was an important member of the new group in much the same way as he had been an important and significant member of the primary school.

By contrast, the middle-class boy who saw the grammar school as the regular next step in his career, had fewer expectations and accepted more readily the large, impersonal school and his own insignificant position in it.

This oversimplified picture highlights the fact that the way in which the school's actions are interpreted depends on the expectations and frame of reference the boy brings to the situation ; in the one case, the large impersonal and somewhat anomic character of a grammar school is taken as something which one has with time to get accustomed to, and which will change ; in the other it is seen as a set of cues to be evaluated as signifying acceptance or indifference.

The situation is more complex than this ; for, as I pointed out at the beginning of the paper, the correlation between social class and leaving age for the country as a whole is only in the order of 0·25.[7] In our sample it was even smaller, although not significantly different.[5] An additional important factor is the school itself. We noticed this factor forcibly when we examined the social class composition of the schools and related these to the percentage of boys who did not enter the sixth form. Using the social class composition of the third form as an index, we can divide the four grammar schools into a predominantly working-class school (school A), one mixed school (school B), and two predominantly middle-class schools (schools C and D). Our findings are tabulated in Table II.

It will be seen that the leaving rate for three out of the four schools was remarkably similar despite the considerable variation in social class composition, especially between schools A, and C and D. To understand more precisely the role of the school, we examined the internal organization of each school ; first, simply by ascertaining how far the pupils in the schools were streamed according to ability, and second, how far such

TABLE II

School	*N*	Percentage of middle- and working-class boys in the 3rd Forms of 4 Grammar Schools		Percentage of boys who left before age of Seventeen
		middle-class	working-class	
A	86	30	70	55
B	70	51	49	57
C	66	59	41	55
D	41	59	41	41
All	263	48	52	53

streaming was stressed by the school and perceived as such by the boys themselves. We found in schools A and B a positive and significant correlation (+0·290) between intelligence test results and stream ; this was not the case in the other two schools.

We have said earlier that the working-class boy, to be induced to stay on, needed success experiences. In the schools which had a clear élite system, success was *assigned* by placing the boys in the top stream: Table III shows the relation of streaming in schools A and B to early leaving.*

From our conversations with the headmasters at the time, we gained the impression that streaming was made a more important feature in school A than in school B. Not only

* The hypotheses about the effect of streaming on leaving age were developed from an examination of the data; their validity would, of course, have to be tested on a new sample. The terms ' achieved ' and ' assigned ' success were coined by D. A. Young.

were the pupils in A streamed by ability, but the teachers more readily conveyed the impression to the boys in the top stream that special things were expected of them. In the light of our hypothesis that the working-class boys will stay only if they have early and tangible experiences of success and that success can be either *assigned* or *achieved*, we postulated that where the organizational structure was strong the relative importance of achieved success would be reduced, and where it was not so strong the importance of achieved success would be enhanced. Inspection of the relative size of correlations

TABLE III

PERCENTAGE OF BOYS IN SCHOOLS A AND B IN EACH OF THE THREE STREAMS WHO LEFT BEFORE THE AGE OF SEVENTEEN

	School A		School B	
Stream	*N*	Per cent early leavers	*N*	Per cent early leavers
A	32	27	27	48
B	21	57	22	68
C	33	85	21	57

between leaving age and the two success indices bears this out (Table IV). The table shows that in school A there was a significant correlation between leaving age and stream (assigned success) ; in school B, between leaving age and self-assessed class position (achieved success). In both these schools, the correlation between early leaving age and father's occupation was not significant.

The school in which streaming operated most strongly was also the school which contained the highest proportion of working-class pupils. It seems that the school responded to the challenge of its intake (whose norm would be to leave rather than stay the course) by creating an élite group within the school itself, thereby ensuring that, even if the school ethos could not touch all the children, a sizeable proportion remained.

W. Brandis carried the analysis a step further by examining the internal structure of the other two grammar schools (C and D), those with a higher proportion of middle- than working-class pupils. Although these schools did not stream by ability (the correlation was −0·172), the comments of the headmaster and, above all, the recollections of the young men suggest that in school D there was a marked system of streaming with a clear cut élite group. (Eighty per cent felt this to be the case.) School D certainly had no 'social class problem', but it did have an ability problem. Table V gives the distribution of IQ ratings for the four schools.

TABLE IV

CORRELATIONS WITHIN SCHOOLS A AND B OF THE BOYS' LEAVING AGE WITH SELF-ASSESSED CLASS POSITION, STREAM AND SOCIAL BACKGROUND

CORRELATION WITH LEAVING AGE	SCHOOL A	SCHOOL B
Stream (assigned success)	+0·583 †	+0·222
Self-assessed class position (achieved success)	+0·043	+0·380 *
Father's occupation	+0·042	+0·174

* Significant at 1 per cent level.
† Significant at 0·01 per cent level.

School D had far fewer pupils of high ability than any of the other schools; yet, after school A, it was the most successful school, judged by the percentage of boys who stayed the course and by those who sat and passed A-level examinations. How was this achieved?

The same pattern emerged as in the case of schools A and B. The stronger the hierarchical system, the less important was self-assessed position in class (achieved success). In school D it was stream which related most strongly to leaving, whereas in school C it was self-assessed form position (Table VI).

The explanation of this lies in the nature of the streaming; it was not, as we have seen, streaming by ability. The conversation with the headmaster showed that, instead, streaming was designed rather to reward hard work. That this was so was shown by the positive correlation between age of leaving and teachers' ratings of the boy's industry at thirteen, a correlation we obtained in school D and in none of the others. Emphasis on the virtues of hard work, on the adequate performance of homework, is necessary if pupils of relatively low ability are to succeed. These are qualities which are

TABLE V

Distribution of Pupils by IQ Ratings in each of the Four Grammar Schools

IQ Rating	School A ($N = 86$) Per cent	School B ($N = 70$) Per cent	School C ($N = 66$) Per cent	School D ($N = 41$) Per cent
122 and over	31	49	39	17
115–122	36	30	29	29
Less than 115	33	21	32	54

TABLE VI

Correlations of Leaving Age with Stream and Self-assessed Form Position and Father's Occupation for Schools C and D

Correlation with Leaving Age of:	School C	School D
Stream	+0·140	+0·418 *
Self-assessed form position	+0·358 *	+0·221
Father's occupation	+0·228	+0·429 *

* Significant at 1 per cent level.

valued also by middle-class families, with their stress on educational achievement, and which these families try to engender in their children. In this school the positive correlation between background and leaving would seem to be a reflection of the ethos of the school ; those who come from middle-class families have already accepted the ethos ; those from working-class backgrounds who respond to it positively, stay the course.

For instance, in the A stream those working-class boys who were not singled out by the teachers as being highly industrious at thirteen, left significantly earlier than their middle-class counterparts (0·002 per cent level of significance). The contrast was striking: 92 per cent of the boys in the A stream who stayed were either middle-class boys or working-class boys with a high rating for hard work ; lack of an assigned success position made 93 per cent of the working-class boys in the C stream leave, irrespective of the teachers' ratings of their behaviour or performance.

In this school, then, there were two interrelated indices of success ; the assigned success position afforded by being in the élite stream and the somewhat less important success position achieved through gaining the teacher's approval for hard work. As in the analysis of school A, so here too we find that these factors operate more strongly on the working-class than on the middle-class pupils.

School A and school D had both adopted successful strategies for dealing with their intake problem. Each had an intake which Brandis describes as ' impaired in one or other of two functional requisites ': school A, in retention through having a large proportion of working-class children with a tendency to leave early ; school D, in level of ability. In both, the characteristic in which the school is deficient is played down and other characteristics stressed. In both, success is bought at a high price, namely by the creation of a negative reference group, an inevitable by-product of the élite system.

A different aspect of the follow-up study illustrates once again the importance of accommodation to intake. With the help of the Home Office, we were able to trace all those boys who had come up before the court, either while at school or subsequently, prior to the second interview. We found that among the five secondary modern schools, one school had a particularly high delinquency rate: 30 per cent of that age group had at one time or other come up against the law compared with 14 per cent for the remainder of the schools. Yet, when we looked at the age at which the delinquencies were committed, we found that in this school, significantly more than in any other, the delinquencies had occurred *after* the boy had left school. What had happened was that the school (being situated in a neighbourhood of shifting populations and of problem families) had accommodated to its intake. It had provided a structure within which the young person could feel secure. Once he left school, the full impact of the neighbourhood and the family was felt. Altogether, social background of the family for secondary modern pupils proved an important factor, not in acquiring educational qualifications while at school, but in seeking further education on leaving school. This was particularly so among pupils of relatively high ability (IQ of 107 and above). Of these, 55 per cent of young men from middle-class homes, 33 per cent of those from skilled, and only 16 per cent of those from unskilled working-class homes acquired some educational qualifications after school.

What I have done so far is to describe how one element of the structure of the types of strategies adopted by the school serves to offset or responds to the particular quality of its intake of pupils. Case studies of this type can generate hypotheses whose validity needs to be tested on a new sample. However, what they do bring out is the importance of looking not at single variables, but at the complex of interacting forces. The study further shows:

1. That the school is a powerful socializing agent, and that both its structure and the teachers' attitudes provide cues to which the pupils respond, the responsiveness depending on the pupil's frames of reference and expectations.

2. That schools that have a deficiency in their intake (either an unduly large proportion of working-class pupils who are likely to leave early or pupils of relatively low ability) may try to counteract this by organizational devices, e.g. streaming aimed at stressing characteristics other than the ones in which the intake is deficient.

3. That streaming has an important effect on motivation. This is an aspect which has perhaps been insufficiently stressed in the past. The motivational effect becomes particularly

important where the next step on the educational ladder is no longer imposed, but depends on the decision of the individual pupil, and where the pupil is in a situation in which, because of his background and set of expectations, the decision is a genuine and not a pseudo one. Further, our follow-up study has shown how important are the consequences of this decision.

4. That it may not be possible to create an effective élite group without giving those excluded the feeling of being failures. How the pupil will react to this situation will depend on his past learning experiences and on the set of expectations engendered by his home background.

What I have described is in the nature of a series of case studies, generating hypotheses concerning the fit between school and child. We are now examining the effect of these strategies on the young man's expectations and attitudes, and are also extending the inquiry to secondary modern schools. Since few secondary modern pupils sat O-level examinations, the comparison will be made here in terms of job choice, vocational attainment and work motivation.

These examples show that we need to carry out educational studies based on complex conceptual models which consider certain characteristics of the child—his ability, his tolerance for stress, etc.—within the framework of a series of socializing experiences, first in the family and later in the school.

To consider intake, structure and attainment is to single out very narrow aspects of the total educational experience. These constitute the tip of the iceberg. Such analysis would be more rewarding if we had more psychologically relevant information about the climate of the school and about the teachers' expectations and attitudes.

The analysis I have outlined is protracted because in each instance we asked not why is this relationship there, but why is it not stronger ; what are the forces in particular situations which reduce its impact. It focuses on deviant cases and on sub-groups.

I have also tried to show the natural history of such an analysis, and the way in which the search for reasons to account for lack of regularity has led to the generation of hypotheses about the effect of particular organizational structures upon the individual and also about the response of the organization to its membership.

The purpose of this paper is to stress the need for interaction analysis. In educational research this is novel; not so in the field of research into hospital or industrial organizations. Because of the regrettable compartmentalization of studies into those to do with children and those to do with adults, those concerned with education and those concerned with industry, there is little carry-over of the findings of one field to the other. It is likely that in schools, too, we have something like Herzberg's [3] two factors operating: the maintenance factors which prevent the worker from experiencing hostility and dissatisfaction and the motivating factors which make him keen and interested in his work.

If we accept, at least as a basis for argument, that complex interaction analysis is needed and that the effect of dealing with deficit in intake will vary depending upon the pupil's norm expectations, certain consequences follow for the strategy of research and for educational planning:

1. As far as the Department of Education is involved, a different method is needed for compiling central and regional statistics in such a way that the child can be related to the school and that information about the school's organizational structure and staff are readily available. Our study suggests, too, that the planning of what statistics should be collected might fruitfully be done in consultation with social scientists.

2. Attention should be concentrated on deviant analysis—on schools or pupils who do not follow the rule ; there is a need for closer study of compensatory or aggravating factors. We should ask whether there is one prescription for success and one for failure, or whether there are varieties of such prescriptions and, further, whether strategies which may have similar effects upon educational attainment may have a differential effect upon the child's self-concept, his expectations about himself as an adult, upon his work motivations, etc.

3. It is important to concentrate on *critical* or *cut off* periods; our data, for instance, have shown that the first two years at grammar school are crucial for the working-class child in developing a sense of identification with the norms of the school.

4. We need to validate the theory suggested by our study that the stronger the structure of the school or, to use Goffman's [2] terminology, the more complete the system, the less do antecedent variables matter.

5. We need to study more closely what happens when the structure ceases to operate. We quoted the example of the young man leaving a school that offers him security and then succumbing to the full force of the neighbourhood. It is here that social action might well be launched.

6. We need to consider the unintended effects of a particular organizational pattern and at the same time to study different patterns of organization. This will become particularly important when we move over to comprehensive schools, where the temptation to create some kind of order can lead to internal barriers as powerful in their impact on the pupils as those which exist at present through segregation at the age of eleven-plus.

Research of the type I have outlined for the future will be costly and time-consuming; it will also require far greater collaboration than exists at present between local educational authorities and social scientists, particularly once we move away from the narrow criterion of educational achievement expressed in examination results to the study of the effect of education on the whole man. An analysis on which we are at present engaged shows that the secondary modern pupil and the man who has had a secondary modern school education is less liberal, more authoritarian and more prejudiced in his outlook than his grammar school counterpart. Why is this so? How far it is tied up with what he brings to the school, his own intellectual calibre and his previous learning experiences; and how far with what the school does to him?

My plea is, then, for studies aimed at a fuller understanding of the effect of the school environment upon the child and for a readiness to move from theory-generating studies not just to theory testing, but also to experiments requiring collaboration between education authorities and social scientists in much the same way as has recently been in operation in the United States in the revision of mathematics and science teaching. There, learning principles provided by psychologists, and a thorough understanding of what amounts to the core principles of the disciplines, provided by the most eminent authorities in the field, were welded together into a novel way of teaching the subject. The results of this new method were then evaluated by educationalists and social scientists.

DISCUSSION

In reply to a questioner who commented on the emergence of delinquency in young people after leaving a school in which the influence had been strong enough to contain delinquent tendencies, and who asked what could be done to achieve a more permanent restraining of the delinquent potential, PROFESSOR HIMMELWEIT said that this finding pointed to the weakness in our provision for young people. The headmaster of a school in a high delinquent area had succeeded well in making his school sufficiently meaningful to the young people to act as a counterweight against the delinquent atmosphere of the neighbourhood. Yet around the age of fourteen to fifteen, towards the end of their school career, boys had begun to outgrow the school and by the time they left they were ready for new experiences and influences. The absence of qualifications, lack of educational attainment, the climate of the neighbourhood, the boredom of unskilled jobs, all contributed to undo the impact of the school. There was a need for individual adults who would take an interest in each boy, establish contact with him well before he left school and then continue to keep in touch with him. The Youth Employment Office, as at present staffed and constituted, might not be appropriate. Young people who received relatively little emotional support from home needed such support, especially at the moment of transition from school to work.

A questioner suggested that, since the child's educational motivation became so difficult to influence later in his school life, there should be much more universal nursery education. Professor Himmelweit said she would like to go further ; just as nursery school education, with its respect for different rates of development, had had a good effect on primary school education, so the time had come for this same approach to infiltrate into secondary schools. There was a need for more flexibility in teaching, and, above all, in the type of contact between teacher and pupil than there was at present. If we were to do much more for the underprivileged in particular, we would have to recognize their hunger for emotional support, for encouragement and for success experiences. Once these needs were satisfied, school work would improve and with it the sense of responsibility of the individual to the community, for which self-confidence is an essential prerequisite.

Asked if she could elaborate on differentiation within schools, Professor Himmelweit said that she had tried to show that such differentiation—for example by streaming—had important consequences, not only on how well children did at school, but also on how willing they were to stay on and work for the various examinations which, in our society as at present constituted, were practically the sole means of access to a wide range of occupations. It was, therefore, not enough to have comprehensive schools ; care must also be taken that within such schools streaming did not create an élite and, with it, a failure group. A delicate balance must be struck. How this was done would vary from school to school. What was clear, however, was that rigid streaming had too many disadvantages to be acceptable. There was need for experimentation with appropriate follow-up.

REFERENCES

1. Douglas, J. W. B. 1964. *The Home and the School.* London. MacGibbon and Kee.

2. Goffman, E. 1963. The presentation of self in everyday life. In *Current Perspectives in Social Psychology.* (Ed. E. P. Hollander and R. G. Hunt.) London. Oxford University Press.
3. Herzberg, F. and Mausner, B. 1962. *The Motivation to Work.* New York. Wiley.
4. Himmelweit, Hilde T. 1963. Socio-economic background and personality. In *Current Perspectives in Social Psychology.* (Ed. E. P. Hollander and R. G. Hunt.) London. Oxford University Press.
5. Himmelweit, Hilde T. 1964. A ten-year follow-up study: its objectives and conceptual framework. Paper read at the Annual Conference of the British Psychological Society, Leicester.
6. Ministry of Education. 1954. *Early Leaving Report.* London. H.M.S.O.
7. Ministry of Education. 1961. *Statistics of Education.* Part 3, *Supplementary.* London. H.M.S.O.
8. Turner, R. H. 1961. Modes of social ascent through education: sponsored and contest mobility. In *Education, Economy and Society.* (Ed. A. H. Halsey, J. Floud and C. A. Anderson.) Glencoe, Minn. Free Press of Glencoe.
9. Warburton, F. W. 1964. Attainment and the school environment. In *Education and Environment.* (Ed. S. Wiseman.) Manchester University Press.
10. Wiseman, S. (Ed.) 1964. *Education and Environment.* Manchester University Press.

INTELLIGENCE TESTING AND COMPREHENSIVE EDUCATION

DOUGLAS PIDGEON
National Foundation for Educational Research

THIS paper is primarily concerned with the impact that intelligence testing has had, and is possibly still having, on the development of the education system in this country. The view is taken that the future social and economic advancement of any society depends overwhelmingly upon the investment it is prepared to make in human capital, or in other words, upon what resources it is prepared to put into and what structure it is prepared to impose upon its education system. What proportion of its total income a country is prepared to invest in its education system is, of course, an important issue but one which lies outside the scope of this paper. Within the limitations imposed by the resources available, however, different structures are possible and it is necessary first to consider what these might be.

While the structure of an education system can be exceedingly complex, in general terms it is the policy adopted that determines what kinds of school will be built and what kinds of children will occupy them. The form this organization takes, and particularly the instructional practices adopted within it, largely depend, however, upon the prevailing philosophy. Two quite different philosophies are distinguishable ; Husén [11], borrowing commonly used terms, has recently referred to these as the 'élitist' and the 'comprehensive'. The main aim of the former is to prepare pupils for the university or for managerial or professional jobs. To do this it is essential to maintain high academic standards and this leads to a system of school organization that is characterized by parallelism, i.e. having academic secondary schools running parallel with other types of school, and selectively. The comprehensive philosophy, on the other hand, is primarily concerned with the education of all children, with no special provision for the academically gifted. Selectivity as a principle is rejected, and the emphasis is on guidance and flexibility of choice within a single type of school.

Such brief descriptions as this fail to convey the essential differences between the two philosophies and the education systems they give rise to ; and, since the concern here is with the part that intelligence tests and their use have played in developing and maintaining both the philosophy and the education system of this country, it is intended to examine these in somewhat greater detail.

In most countries of Western Europe, and typically in England, educational systems developed from within highly stratified class societies ; and, possibly because self-preservation is a predominant instinct in man, the systems produced resulted in a maintenance of the existing social structures. Thus, at the end of the nineteenth century in England secondary education was reserved for a privileged élite and was academic in nature with heavy leanings towards the classics. The newer grammar schools set up and maintained by local authorities following the Education Act of 1902 largely followed this tradition, and thus the pattern of what was implied by ' secondary education ' became in time firmly established. In the early decades of the twentieth century, however, began the rise of the intelligence-testing movement and with it confirmation of the opinion that all children were not born intellectually equal. Here then was justification—if indeed it was needed—for giving this secondary education to an élite ; not now a socially privileged or moneyed élite, but an intellectual élite ostensibly drawn from all walks of life.

This, in theory at least, embodied the doctrine of equal opportunity for all. Children were not equal in the extent to which they were capable of absorbing education, but they could all be given the opportunity to receive the highest education unless barred by lack of ability alone. This conception of essential differences amongst children clearly dominated the Hadow and Spens Reports of the thirties which advocated the three types of secondary school—Grammar, Technical, and Modern—and the Norwood Report which discovered that three types of children could be distinguished requiring for the satisfaction of their needs exactly the three kinds of secondary education that had previously been envisaged. Incidentally the Norwood Report went on to say that the assignment of children to the three groups could not necessarily be made with certainty when the children reached the end of their primary school course ; and it suggested that there should be a period between the ages of eleven and thirteen devoted to systematic diagnoses of children's educational needs and capacities in order to allocate them to the most appropriate type of course—a recommendation that foreshadowed the 'observation stage' (*cycle d'observation*) now being implemented some twenty years later in some schools in France and Germany. Unfortunately, little attention was paid to this particular recommendation at the time.

That children differed in their basic ability was a dominant feature of the élitist philosophy. It is intersting to speculate on what would have happened to that philosophy if the work of Galton, Binet, Spearman, Burt and many others had demonstrated that children inherited essentially the same intelligence and that apparent differences in their ability were entirely due to environmental factors amenable to influence by agencies of the educational system. Is it conceivable that the tripartite system would have emerged as it did ? That children would have been separated into different schools and classes and given different kinds and levels of education ? Or that the attitudes of teachers to backward or retarded pupils would have remained the same ? Social traditions would not have been swept away overnight, of course, but if differences in performance had been shown to be due largely to motivational factors inspired by social aspirations, could they have survived for long ?

There is of course overwhelming evidence that the premise on which this speculation is based is false ; yet it serves to stress this basic tenet of the élitist philosophy, namely that since children are different in respect of the abilities they possess, it is necessary to treat them differently. In practice, therefore, so far as the structure of an education system is concerned, the important question is one of grouping. Children must of necessity be grouped into schools and into classes within schools;

and if children of differing abilities require different kinds and levels of education, it is clearly necessary to group them so that these differences are recognized, and the system so arranged that the brightest are successfully steered into appropriate secondary and tertiary courses of education. As Burt [3] has said, " Children of high inborn ability are so scarce that it is the bounden duty of every education authority to ensure that none of them slips unnoticed through the mesh, but that all are caught at the earliest possible age ".

But to be able to do this and to group children according to their inborn ability and to operate an efficient selective system, necessitates the accurate measurement of that ability. Clearly, if it were possible to measure at an early age the innate potential of all children, then, provided the measuring instruments could be refined sufficiently, accurate prediction would present no problem. Once the intellectual capabilities of every child were known, his place in the education system could be readily determined, and errors of selection would be minimal. Moreover, if a child was found not to be working up to his potential, it would be known that the cause was to be found in environmental factors and these could be investigated systematically and appropriate corrective steps taken. Moreover, selection in a competitive system must be made solely on the basis of ability, if equality of opportunity is to have any real meaning. If economic and social factors influence the grouping and hence the selective process, the system falls down on the very factor it stresses as important. Yates [17], summarizing an international conference on grouping practices, has commented recently, " Rigid forms of grouping—the organization of different types of secondary school or the provision of distinct streams or tracks within schools—were clearly defensible when it could be assumed that intellectual potential was largely determined by hereditary factors and could be accurately assessed at a fairly early age ".

There is no need here to reiterate the considerable body of evidence that, over the past twenty years or so, has led to a substantially revised conception of intelligence and to the view that measures of ability are influenced in no minor way by circumstances of children's upbringing and by the quality and duration of their formal education. Referring to this changed conception of intelligence, however, Yates continues, " In these circumstances the early segregation of pupils on the basis of apparent differences in intellectual capacity, especially when this involves according different kinds of educational treatment to the groups so formed, is scarcely justifiable ".

Whether a system of ability-grouping is defensible or not, the point to be made here is that, through the early beliefs about the measurement of innate ability and the continued use of intelligence tests by teachers and administrators, the élitist philosophy has come to be accepted almost without question. Indeed, it seems possible that the majority of teachers and educational administrators, if they are aware that an alternative philosophy exists, have considerable misconceptions about its aims and intentions. This may well be because under the comprehensive philosophy the educational structure is necessarily related to the social structure. This is not to say that research evidence from the sociologists has had no impact, but in the debate now proceeding concerning possible changes in our educational system, the implications are seen in a purely educational context. Husén [11] has suggested that secondary school teachers in particular are suffering from a professional disease which causes them to overlook the fact that a school operates in a social and economic context and that its goals and modes of operation are substantially affected by the changes that are occurring in our present day society.

The acceptance of a given philosophy, of course, is reflected in the attitudes adopted ; and it is in developing and fostering these attitudes that beliefs about intelligence and its measurement, it is claimed, have played a significant part. In particular, the ideas that teachers develop concerning how much, or how little, their pupils are capable of performing are affected in no small measure by the beliefs they hold. Many teachers, for example, are convinced that French can be taught only to children above a certain level of ability. That the attitudes of teachers play an important part in determining the attainments of pupils, has, of course, been recognized [2, 4, 8], but direct research evidence that there is a relation between what teachers expect from their pupils and what they actually achieve would appear to be lacking. In other words, the hypothesis that the standard or level of achievement reached by any group of pupils is dependent upon the standard or level expected of them, has not been subjected to experimental verification. Yet it is possible to cite instances where the assumption of such a relation is in accord with discovered facts. The findings of the *Early Leaving* Report [14], for example, that the proportion of pupils obtaining a ' good ' GCE ' O ' Level result bears no relation to the proportion entering Grammar schools in different parts of the country, may be due in part to the adoption of different standards by examining boards ; but it is also possible that some teachers expect, and obtain, results that others do not. One may question also whether the superior performances of boys over girls in mathematics is not also due, in part at least, to the generally accepted belief that this is a ' boys' ' subject and girls cannot be expected to do as well.

It is in the area of ability grouping, however, that this notion of expectancy could—and it is suggested, does—operate markedly ; for it is here that the teacher's beliefs about the education system in which he is working predominate. A teacher who firmly believes that children's education should be matched to their abilities, as, of course, is implied by the 1944 Education Act, is much more likely to underestimate than overestimate what they are really capable of doing. The teacher of a ' B ' stream, for example, clearly expects a rather lower level of performance from his pupils than the teacher of an ' A ' stream ; and in general he gets it—though there is, of course, always a considerable overlap. It is questionable, however, whether the lower performance obtained from the ' B ' stream pupils is entirely due to their lower ability. As Douglas [5] and others have shown, the ' B ' stream is likely to be over-represented with children from manual working-class homes, for whom any measure of their potential (whether made by test or by judgement) will be an underestimate. Thus, even if the teacher is successful in getting them to work to the limits of their apparent capacity, their performances will fall short of what may be presumed to be theoretically possible.

Unfortunately, however, the view that the teacher gets is

likely to convince him that his outlook is right, for the so-called self-fulfilling prophecy works here, and the more successful he is in matching his pupils' attainments to their abilities, the more successful will any initial streaming appear to be. Yates [17] refers to the same point when he says, " The prediction of relative success or failure, even when based on psychometrically dubious procedures, is often borne out in practice, largely because children are obliging creatures and are inclined to produce the standard of work that their elders regard as appropriate ".

The argument adopted here applies with equal, if not greater, force to the separation of pupils into Grammar and Modern schools, and it can be used to illustrate the point that the élitist philosophy is self-perpetuating. Teachers who have themselves been through the selective system, have been trained to teach in it, and inevitably see it as succeeding, are not generally disposed to become its critics. They may be aware of its fallibility, but they see the faults as either inevitable or capable of correction, and do not question the assumptions on which it is based.

Nevertheless, changes in our education system are being made. There is a definite trend away from streaming in primary schools, and comprehensive schools at the secondary level are being built. These, however, are changes in structure only and in all too rare instances are they accompanied or preceded by changes in the attitudes of teachers. Research now being carried out on the question of streaming in primary schools would suggest that in many large non-streamed schools pupils are still fairly rigidly grouped for ability within their class, and in only a few is it clear that élitist attitudes to children's capabilities have been completely rejected.

There is probably a greater loosening of attitudes within primary than within secondary schools, however. Marklund [12] found that in Sweden the specialist subject teachers at the secondary level had a more negative attitude than primary class teachers to the policy of reform aimed at introducing comprehensive education. Although a full-scale survey of comprehensive schools has not yet been made, what little evidence there is would suggest that there are few that do not stream and probably fewer where the consequences for teachers of accepting the comprehensive philosophy have been fully appreciated, and appropriate action taken. It would seem that, with one or two possible exceptions, it is the physical organization alone that characterizes a comprehensive school in England. That is to say, any school in which it is the aim to have pupils of all ranges of ability and from all sections of the community represented, is regarded as comprehensive regardless of its internal structure. Thus, even if children of all ranges of ability are taught within one school, they may be given very different kinds of education, according to whether they are considered suitable for an academic course, or only for a more general or practical one ; and even within such courses, they may be rigidly streamed for ability. Research carried out so far has been rather limited and generally confined to a study of only one or two schools. The findings of Miller [13] suggest that the secondary modern type of pupil would seem to gain, from the cultural, social and educational point of view, by being in a comprehensive school ; but the studies of Dixon,[4] Futcher [6] and Holly [10] suggest that the streaming structure adopted does little to bring about the greater social unification which presumably is one of the intended aims.

What kind of structure is envisaged under the comprehensive philosophy ? It is seen as essentially one in which the grouping of children in terms of their apparent abilities must be eschewed ; for to group them so will inevitably result in differentiation by social and cultural factors also, thus preventing the realization of the aim of equality of opportunity. An education system must be seen in its social context, however, and if the aim is to minimize social differences in society, this will be achieved only by ensuring that the pupils are grouped in school in such a way as to maximize these differences within the groups. There would appear to be a general principle here, that using a factor as a basis of grouping and making groups homogeneous with respect to it, tends to maximize its effect in society. Grouping based on distinctions of race or religion, for example, helps to emphasize or even exaggerate these distinctions.

This would certainly seem to be true with respect to ability and achievement. It has been contended elsewhere that dividing children into groups homogeneous for ability results in a gradual widening of the differences in performance between the brightest and the dullest. Many comparative studies have shown [1, 7] that the variability in performance of children is consistently greater in England than in the United States, where in general heterogeneous ability grouping is practised.

The comprehensive philosophy, of course, requires rather more than the acceptance of the principle of heterogeneous grouping by ability or social factors. In effect, it also requires considerably less emphasis on individual differences in ability, while at the same time stressing the need for individual guidance. This seems to present something of a dilemma. If cognizance is not to be taken of ability differences within the class group, for example, does this mean that all children are to be given the same instruction regardless of ability? Such a procedure is in direct antithesis to the élitist conception that children do differ in ability and to teach them all together will necessarily result in both the bright and the dull suffering; and it has been argued here that, if teachers expect that some children in their class will not do as well as they might, then this expectation will materially influence the children's actual performances.

It is clearly unnecessary, however, to assume that giving the same instruction to all children regardless of ability is either the only or even the correct solution to an acceptance of the comprehensive philosophy. Indeed, the evidence is fairly conclusive that children are not born equally gifted intellectually, and it would be just as wrong to assume they were as to assume that observed or measured abilities gave an accurate reflection of innate differences. But to recognize that differences can exist without assuming that they correspond to the observed differences in performance at any given time and without over-emphasizing their importance, requires not only a differential attitudinal approach but also the application of different teaching methods. Inevitably, full acceptance of the comprehensive philosophy will demand individualization, i.e. an educational structure which emphasizes individual learning and utilizes such modern conceptions as programmed learning and team teaching, and such technological advances as language laboratories, television, looped-film projectors and teaching machines.

The comprehensive philosophy, therefore, demands that teachers become aware not only of the social implications of the school and of the functions of education in a changing society, but also of their own changing role in the learning process. Its acceptance will thus have repercussions, not only on grouping practices, on curriculum construction and on instructional practices in the classroom, but also on teacher training and in-service training. Moreover, the abolition of a selective system will have implications for our present conception of university education.

Intelligence tests may have had their usefulness in the selective system, though it has been argued here that their function has been largely that of justifying that system and then of perpetuating it. In a comprehensive system, on the other hand, where emphasis is to be placed on individual guidance and on the substitution of elective rather than selective courses in the later stages of secondary education, it is difficult to see what place they will have. Tests may possibly be developed which will provide descriptions of many different kinds of intelligent behaviour; but if the view—expressed in the foreword to the Newsom Report [15]—that intelligence can be acquired represents current thinking, then the results of even such tests will have no permanent significance for pupil guidance.

Clearly, however, there is a need here for research. Indeed, if guidance is to be given to the administrators, curriculum developers, teachers and others who will operate in a system of comprehensive education, a great deal of research will be necessary. It is important, however, that such research be carried out within the context of the comprehensive philosophy, and not just in schools which may be *called* comprehensive, but in which the attitudes and beliefs of the existing system still predominate.

REFERENCES

1. Anderson, I. H. 1964. *Comparisons of the Reading and Spelling Achievement and Quality of Handwriting of Groups of English, Scottish and American Children.* Co-operative Research Project No. 1903. University of Michigan.
2. Bachus, M. K. 1959. *A Survey of the Secondary Modern Teachers' Concepts of their Pupils' Interests and Abilities in relation to their Social Philosophy and to the Social Class Background of their Pupils.* Unpublished M.A. Thesis University of London.
3. Burt, C. 1959. General ability and special aptitudes. *Educ. Res.* **1**, 2.
4. Dixon, S. 1962. *Some Aspects of Social Life and Progress in a Comprehensive School in Relation to Pupils' Social Background.* M.A. Thesis University of London.
5. Douglas, J. W. B. 1964. *The Home and the School.* London. MacGibbon and Kee.
6. Futcher, W. G. 1960. *A Comparative Study of Attitudes and Personality Traits of Children in Certain Comprehensive, Grammar and Modern Schools in London.* M.A. Thesis, London.
7. Gibson, R. L. 1965. *A Comprehensive Study of the Academic Achievements of Elementary Age Students of the United States and the British Isles.* U.S.O.E. Project No. 2177. University of Toledo.
8. Goodacre, E. 1965. *Teachers' Attitudes to their Pupils' Home Background.* Ph.D. Thesis, University of London.
9. Himmelweit, Hilde T. 1955. Socio-economic background and personality. *Unesco International Social Science Bulletin,* **7**, 1.
10. Holly, D. H. 1963. *The Structure and Functioning of a London Comprehensive School.* M.A. Thesis, University of London.
11. Husén, T. *The Contribution of Research to the Reform of Secondary Education.* Paper presented to the Quadrennial Congress of the International Association for the Advancement of Educational Research.
12. Marklund, S. 1963. The attitude of intending teachers to school reform in Sweden. In *Yearbook of Education* 1963.
13. Miller, T. W. G. 1958. *A Critical and Empirical Study of the Imagined Development and Significance of the Comprehensive Secondary School in England with Special Reference to Certain Educational and Social Effects.* Ph.D. Thesis, University of Birmingham.
14. Ministry of Education. 1954. *Early Leaving.* Report of the Central Advisory Council for Education. London. H.M.S.O.
15. Ministry of Education. 1964. *Half our Future.* Report of the Central Advisory Council for Education (England). London. H.M.S.O.
16. Pidgeon, D. A. 1962. A comparative study of the dispersions of test scores. In *Educational Achievements of Thirteen Year Olds in Twelve Countries.* Unesco Institute for Education. Hamburg.
17. Yates, A. 1966. *Grouping in Education.* Unesco Institute for Education, Hamburg.

SELECTION FOR HIGHER EDUCATION

Chairman : Lord Robbins

PRINCIPLES AND PROCEDURES OF UNIVERSITY SELECTION

JEAN FLOUD
Nuffield College, Oxford

THERE are important scientific and technical problems underlying the art of educational selection and guidance : for example, the nature-nurture controversy, and how to assess motivation as well as talent. But I think that the political and administrative problems involved in selection are just as important and almost equally difficult. In case they should be overlooked in our discussions I propose to say something about them—perhaps to overstate them in order to right the balance—in a gathering of scientists, who may be inclined to underestimate their importance.

We know extraordinarily little about the validity of the different procedures used in university selection ; but more important than our ignorance, it seems to me, is our tendency, when faced with the unavoidable necessity of selecting, to misconceive the real nature of the activity itself and to allow ourselves to be diverted from consideration of its intrinsically political and procedural or administrative character. We readily slip into a frame of mind in which we tacitly assume a theory of academic predestination, imagining ourselves to be faced with a scientific problem of predicting and a technical problem of competitive elimination, whereas it would be nearer the truth, I think, to see ourselves as faced with a political problem of choice or election, and an administrative or procedural problem of ways and means.

If we were starting from scratch to devise an admissions system, it would have to be in the light of the three general criteria by which we judge existing systems and find them lacking : we should want our admissions system to be at one and the same time academically successful, educationally defensible, and socially just in its outcome. I propose to consider what is involved in applying each of these criteria.

(I shall have no time to carry the matter further and argue the case for its being academically enterprising, educationally constructive and socially progressive.)

To be *academically successful* a university needs to compete efficiently with others in attracting promising students of the right age and maturity for tackling difficult honours courses. This means drawing without impediment, on equal terms with others, on the largest possible population of potential candidates—namely, the total of boys and girls of seventeen and over in the Sixth Forms of all the secondary schools in the country. So much is indisputable ; the question is, how will efficiency show itself? One might argue that it will show in two ways : (1) in top-heavy class lists, with next to no failures and buoyant contingents of Firsts and good Seconds ; (2) in sound predictions about the performance of those admitted (holders of Scholarships should do conspicuously well ; those accepted reluctantly should do less well than those accepted with alacrity ; we should feel confident that among those rejected there are few or none who would have done as well as those admitted).

However, this argument rests on the assumption that the efficiency of selection techniques can be judged by the accuracy with which they enable us to predict the performance of candidates in the final examinations ; the better the tests, the higher the probability of an accurate forecast. But Professor Drever [2] has shown convincingly that this is a profoundly misleading assumption, for the fundamental reason that many of the factors relevant to the future performance of candidates are not merely indeterminate, but indeterminable and beyond the reach of any improvement in forecasting devices. Here, I think, one must have in mind not merely strictly random factors such as " an inspiring teacher, a pretty face, a subject encountered for the first time " [2], but, much more important, the indeterminable outcome of the higher educational process itself, with its multiple, confused objectives and its largely intuitive and unselfconscious use of traditional teaching methods deriving from the idea of the university as an academic Guild with its masters, journeymen and apprentices. The truth is, as Professor Drever showed in his lecture, that, over a wide field of applications between the obviously outstanding and the patently unqualified, we are simply not in a position to apply the competitive principle. However good our examining or testing, we cannot eliminate ' predictor uncertainty ', which is intrinsic to the problem of university selection ; and within the broad zones of predictor uncertainty we are electing not selecting, choosing not predicting. But on what principles, within this zone of the academically indistinguishable, should we make the choice or election ? This is the area of doubt and debate in respect of which the universities are driven by to-day's pressure on places, to formulate policy. The question is, in fact, a political one : what kind of an academic community are we, or do we want to be ? No university can evade the problem by taking refuge in the complexities of a misconceived meritocratic problem—in the technicalities of teaching and examining, or psycho-genetic questions of environment and heredity as factors in the determination of ability.

In this country and in America the idea of a university as an academic community, a society of scholars, is the natural touchstone of admissions policy. The desire to sustain a variety of types, to produce a balanced community, is everywhere very strong, and particularly so in the small and moderate-sized institutions like the Oxford and Cambridge Colleges, Harvard College and the American Liberal Arts Colleges. These are all self-contained and self-conscious communities, sensitive to the non-academic claims of candidates and well placed—confronted as they mostly are with relatively small numbers—to discover and assess these. But no one can ignore the competitive element in admissions to-day ; it is a fact of life for the universities. Hence there is often a feeling of guilt about the search for a balanced academic community which, it is supposed, will involve a sacrifice of efficiency, if not actual injustice in selection. If weight is given to non-academic considerations in choosing candidates, it is argued, the order of merit is violated. But, as we have seen, this is to confuse something that certainly can happen and no doubt does take place in practice with the inherent nature of the problem, which is different. The strict ' order of merit ' is an illusion :

the broad zones of 'predictor uncertainty', the nature and force of the educative environment are the reality.

When Sir Maurice Bowra [1] gave evidence recently to the Franks Commission of Inquiry into the University of Oxford, he declared: "The best candidates are those who will gain most from what a college offers, and this is the fundamental principle of selection". It is difficult to see how this dictum could be put to the test; like any good educational argument it involves a self-defeating as well as a self-fulfilling prophecy. Not only do we select the best and see that they do as well as they should, but, to the extent that we select effectively on Sir Maurice Bowra's fundamental principle, many candidates will necessarily do better than would be predicted from their performance in the entrance examination.

The basic problems, then, are of a political and administrative character; the scientific and technical problems are necessarily subordinate and for the most part they are not susceptible to very rigorous treatment. Each university must ask itself these questions: What do we claim to offer students—what is our special excellence? What, in the conditions of to-day, constitutes a balanced community? How shall we secure, by the same token, a balanced entry? How shall we decide, given our special excellence, for whom we can do most? If, choosing on this principle from amongst a balanced entry, we find ourselves confronted with an unrepresentative intake, what is the remedy? Is the remedy in our own hands? What is the cost, in terms of our aims and identity, of a balanced intake? Are we to regard it as an overriding objective?

The requirement that an admissions system should "*have results that are socially just*" [3] is not a new one in the history of British and American universities, but the scope and implications of the requirement have grown out of recognition in both countries since 1945. The stipulation of social justice is the principal key to the notion of a balanced community in present-day universities and its first condition is the same as for academic success: namely, free and equal access to the national pool of would-be entrants to the universities. It will not do merely to establish formal equality of treatment as between all who actually present themselves for admission; the opportunity of applying must be extended as widely as possible and, in selecting, allowances must be made for differences and inequalities between homes and schools which impose handicaps on particular classes of candidate. Equality of opportunity in this sense would result in an intake of students socially representative at least of the university-going population as a whole. Some would argue for more radical measures which would make the student body socially representative of a wider population—say, of the Sixth Forms of the secondary schools, or even of the age-group as a whole—but this takes us outside the province of an admissions system into the main stream of educational and social policy and raises wider issues than are relevant to this discussion.

There is no incompatibility, in principle, between the aims of social justice in the ordinary sense of equality of opportunity and effective competition for talent. The university should recruit proportionately at least as many working-class students as there are boys and girls of this class coming forward to the universities from the Sixth Forms of the secondary schools; this can be achieved by seeing to it that applications come from the different types of secondary school in proportions closely resembling those in which university candidates are distributed among them, and that the same percentage, more or less, of the total of applications from each type of school is admitted. But there are difficulties here. It is doubtful whether a policy of social justice in university selection can rest itself to-day on differences in the grant-earning status of schools. We aim at social justice because we want to be fair to individuals, and the largest class of educationally handicapped individuals is drawn from working-class families. But it is perfectly possible, in to-day's circumstances, to achieve an intake of students which is properly representative of the different types of school (maintained, direct grant, and independent), which reflects the social composition of the university-going population as a whole, but which is nevertheless unfair in its incidence on individuals and in consequence unrepresentative of the distribution of talent.

This possibility arises from a combination of circumstances.

The pressure of competition has so raised the level of achievement necessary to secure a university place that success is increasingly dependent on being able and willing to stay on at school into the third year of the Sixth Form. In most schools this acts for most pupils more as an incentive to reach the Sixth Form early—by an ' express route ' through the middle school—than to stay on longer at school. Yet many maintained schools find it difficult and wasteful of their teaching resources to provide a third year in the Sixth Form for the small minority of their pupils who will go on to a university. A growing number of schools, and in particular most girls' schools, also take the view that the curtailed main-school course which is the price of an extended Sixth Form course is, in any case, educationally undesirable, if not in itself, then for the kind of pupil for whom they largely cater. Then there is the reorganization of the secondary schools along comprehensive lines : the many schemes involving a change of school at thirteen rather than eleven may well make it difficult to bring pupils to the level of university entry by the age of eighteen which is, for most of them, and certainly for the girls, the latest age at which they will wish to remain at school or to which the local authorities will be willing to keep them there.

In effect, therefore, the relevant distinctions today are not as between types but as between size and organization of school. Big selective schools, whether maintained, direct grant or independent, can build up third year Sixth Forms for university entrants ; small or non-selective schools find this too difficult, or they may regard it as undesirable anyway ; moreover, many of these schools are in the North and all of them draw most of their entry from the working class.

The maintained schools are more representative socially than other types of school but they do not form an educationally homogeneous group. The number of schools with Sixth Forms producing candidates for university entry is large and growing fast ; but the number offering a third year, or even a seventh term, of advanced work in the Sixth Form and an accelerated stream to O-level is much smaller and growing much more slowly. No admissions policy will be fair and efficient which neglects these vital differences within the maintained sector in the pace at which pupils are brought to the Sixth Form and the amount of ground they can have covered by the time they present themselves for admission to the university. All candidates must have a reasonable chance to demonstrate the intellectual promise for which the university is looking, regardless of differences beyond their control in the organization of their secondary school course.

To be *educationally defensible* an admissions system must not be such as to disrupt relations with other universities or with the schools. The interests of all universities are essentially the same and the interests of the universities generally do not differ from those of the schools. There must be no unfair competition for talent, no arbitrary elements in the timing or conditions of admission, no special entrance examination of a kind that can be shown to exert a bad influence on school curricula or to distort the allocation of resources or the organization of teaching against the interests of the bulk of pupils who do not proceed to higher education. Stated in this general form, these principles do not appear difficult to apply. In practice, however, they could only be applied to the admissions system of a particular university in the context of a general reform of the national system.

The pressure on schools of present arrangements for admission to the universities is notorious and comes in the main from the use of the A-level examination for selection purposes. This is designed to be a leaving examination, intended to record achievement in the work of the past two or three years. Misused by the universities as an entrance examination in a highly competitive situation, it gives rise to the narrow and repetitive teaching in the Sixth Form about which complaint is so often heard. In a growing number of schools the seventh term in the Sixth Form is a mere repetition of the fourth in order to improve the A-level performance of pupils who have secured university places conditional upon their obtaining better grades this year than last.

The Crowther Committee's unqualified indictment of the use of A-levels for purposes of university selection has gone unheeded and the present national admissions system is defensible from the point of view of neither the schools nor the universities, based as it is on performance at a school leaving examination which is a test of performance rather than promise, and which most candidates have not yet sat when their applications are under consideration by the universities of their choice. Only Oxford and Cambridge with their special entrance examinations, taken in the majority of instances after A-levels, stand outside this system. Their arrangements are open to many objections and they fail on various counts in relation to the criteria I have been discussing ; but it is difficult to see how they can be effectively reformed without radical review of the national system. The schools need to be rescued from the grind of competitive grades at A-level and cannot be asked to endure the still greater competitive pressure and the removal of all incentive to post-A-level work in the Sixth Form which would result from the abandonment of the Oxbridge special entrance examinations. The universities need special entrance tests of their own devising suitable to candidates from every type of Sixth Form, and they stand to gain nothing from reinforcement, by the entry of Oxbridge, of the existing irrational national arrangements.

It is clearly in the interests of everyone, and not least of the candidates themselves, that the system should be overhauled. A number of possible reforms come to mind, of which the most radical would involve the universities setting up a testing organization of their own, perhaps on lines similar to those developed in America under the auspices of the College Entrance Board. On the face of it there seems to be no reason why A-levels should not be retained for matriculation purposes whilst candidates are chosen on the basis of their performance in scholastic aptitude and achievement tests in conjunction with school records and possibly an essay or general paper as well. Such arrangements would have the minimum of disruptive effect on the schools and would leave the field free in the universities for experiment with techniques and procedures of selection.

Of course, schemes of this kind set us on the American road, which looks from over here rather like a slippery slope. We have been warned ! A correspondent of the *New Yorker* recently remarked, ". . . the once fairly placid business of college admissions has lately acquired the dimensions of a sizeable industry, some of the jargon of social science, and a structure like that of a vertically organized labour union ". But, as I have said, the problems of university admission are as much political and administrative as technical ; we must rely therefore on rules of good sense.

REFERENCES

1. Bowra, Sir M. 1966. *Written Evidence to Commission of Inquiry into Oxford University*, Part IV, p. 18. London. Oxford University Press.
2. Drever, J. 1963. *Godfrey Thomson Memorial Lecture*. London. Oxford University Press.
3. Robbins Committee. 1963. *Report on Higher Education*, para. 217. London. H.M.S.O. Cmnd. 2154.

ENVIRONMENTAL AND INNATE FACTORS AND EDUCATIONAL ATTAINMENT

STEPHEN WISEMAN
School of Education, University of Manchester

THE organization of this Conference, and the shape which it has taken, is symptomatic of the surge of interest in what is usually called 'educational sociology', an interest which is certainly not confined to the ranks of the professionals—the sociologists and psychologists, the teachers and the teacher trainers. The relationship between social class and educational opportunity, the iniquities of eleven-plus selection, the comprehensive school—these form the talking points not only in school staff rooms and meetings of educationists, but also in the railway carriage and over the coffee table. There is now a general awareness that the educational system and the social system cannot be separated, that they interpenetrate and interact; a general suspicion that, though our overall objectives may be reasonably correct, there is a serious mis-match in the organizations of the two systems. The involvement of such matters with political thought and political belief is obvious, and inescapable. And this leads to the inevitably exaggerated attitudes on both wings, the overemphasis of some facts and factors and the playing-down of others, the introjection of emotive description and propaganda techniques. All this makes it the more important—and the more difficult—to set out soberly and dispassionately what we *know* about the educational-social interaction, rather than to proclaim what we *believe*.

And what we know is precious little. We have only just begun to tease out one or two of the significant strands in what is an enormously complex fabric: the time for certainty is still far away. Most work has been done on the connections between environmental factors—mainly social class—and educational opportunity rather than educational attainment. It is not my intention to consider this part of the field, but merely to note its importance in demonstrating the existence of a major problem, and in acting as a motivator for further work.

The first significant attack in this country on the school environment and its relation to attainment was that of Kemp in 1955.[12] He studied fifty primary schools in London, identifying twenty-eight environmental variables (subsequently pooled to make twelve) and two criteria of attainment: comprehension, and rote-learning. His main conclusions were: (1) that the main factors determining level of attainment in the formal school subjects are, in decreasing order of importance, intelligence, socio-economic status, and size of school; and (2) that progressiveness, new buildings and class size are little (though positively) related to level of attainment. In 1956, Mollenkopf[15] in the USA reported a study of 18,000 ninth and twelfth grade pupils in 206 schools. He concluded: " As was expected, the IQ of the students predicted the achievement test means considerably better (0·90) than did the best-weighted composite of school, parent and community characteristics (0·59). Yet some characteristics did add to the effectiveness of this prediction. Among these were the percentages of graduates going on to college, the size of the average instructional class, and the presence or absence of a community library ".

The results of these two researches are hardly epoch-making, nor do they throw much light on the school factors important for scholastic success. It will be noted that intelligence comes out as the supreme determinant of achievement in both inquiries. No doubt, you will say, this is because of its well-known dependence on socio-economic status. Kemp, however, investigated this particular aspect of his results. His comprehension variables correlated 0·73 with intelligence. " However," he says, " it must be noted that socio-economic status is correlated very significantly with both intelligence (0·52) and this kind of attainment (0·56). When socio-economic status is partialled out the correlation (of 0·73) drops to 0·62. If *intelligence* is held constant, the correlation between socio-economic status and attainment drops (from 0·56) to 0·30. The influence of socio-economic status on attainment appears thus to be much less powerful than that of intelligence." A similar result was obtained with his measures of rote attainment.

During the past decade we have carried out four surveys in the Manchester district, in which we have endeavoured to lay bare some of the associations between environmental factors and educational attainment. Three of these have already been described in detail in *Education and Environment* (1964) [17] and I do not propose to dwell on these, except in so far as they bear on particular matters discussed later. The fourth—an investigation of forty-four primary schools—has just been completed, and although the analyses are not yet finished, some interesting and suggestive results are already to hand. One feature of the Manchester surveys which differentiates them from other researches in this field is the use of measures of backwardness and brightness as well as of average score. All our surveys have used the school as a unit, and we have calculated the percentage of 'bright' and of 'backward' children in each school (using these terms as a shorthand for describing these scoring more than 1 SD above the mean on a particular test, and those scoring less than 1 SD below). All four surveys demonstrate conclusively that brightness and backwardness are not just simple opposites, that some social factors correlate significantly with one and not with the other, and vice versa. It is curious that other researchers have not shown more interest in investigating this aspect of the environment-attainment interaction. Burt [5] in 1943 reported 'decidedly higher' correlations with environmental factors for brighter children than for duller; Fraser (1959) [9] found a significant relationship between ability level and the effect of abnormal home background, with the brighter children being more affected; while Maxwell (1953) [13] concluded from the results of the 1947 Scottish Mental Survey that 'high intellectual ability is more widely distributed over different social environments than is low intellectual ability'. Our own results fall into line with this general trend: brightness has higher correlations with environmental factors than does backwardness. We shall return to this point later.

Our sample of forty-four primary schools was a random

one, stratified by school type (county, C of E, RC) and by area of the city. We concentrated on the 10+ pupils, who had been longest in school. For these pupils we had standardized test results at four ages: 7+, 8+, 9+ and 10+, on tests of intelligence, English and arithmetic, so that we were able to look at age-trends. There were twelve tests altogether (two at 7, three at 8, two at 9 and five at 10), and each test gave us three 'scores' for each school (mean score, per cent bright and per cent backward) so we had thirty-six criterion variables. In addition to this we had fifty-two environmental variables, eighteen relating to the home and the neighbourhood, thirty-four relating to the school itself—its buildings, its equipment, its teachers and its atmosphere. This gave us a total of eighty-eight variables and a matrix of 3828 correlations. The factor analysis of this is not yet completed, but I can report on the chief results from the intercorrelations.

Perhaps the easiest way of summarizing the data is to calculate the average correlation of each environmental variable with all the thirty-six test variables (making appropriate sign adjustments, since the signs for backwardness and brightness are in opposite directions). A stronger connection is found with the social factors in the home and neighbourhood than with the school variables. This is shown if we average the correlations of all the eighteen social variables with the total tests. The result, 0·295, contrasts sharply with a similar average for the thirty-four school variables, 0·199. It seems as if the forces operating outside the school walls are more pervasive and more powerful than those within. The highest correlations underline the factors of *poverty* and *maternal care* that we found in our previous surveys with secondary school children:

Per cent verminous children	0·48
Cleanliness of home	0·48
Per cent free meals	0·47
Material needs inadequate	0·44
Parental occupation	0·42
Family crime	0·38

The highest 'school' correlations are:

Appearance and sociability of children	0·42
Attendance	0·41
Streaming	0·39

The first of these three measures is probably wrongly placed, and ought to be included amongst the 'home' variables; no doubt the school may have some effect here, but the home is almost certainly the major influence. The second on the list—attendance—is a logical result, though many might have expected a higher correlation. The third variable, streaming, is one of particular topical interest. Our results show that streamed schools have *better* records of attainment. As might be expected, the highest individual correlations are with our measures of brightness: brightness, 10+ Composition, 0·66; brightness, 10+ Arithmetic I, 0·60; brightness, 9+ English, 0·60. But there is no suggestion that streaming has an adverse effect on the children of low ability: streamed schools tend to have fewer backward children at all ages and in all tests. It is possible, however, that the association between streaming and attainment is an artifact, since many of our unstreamed schools were one-form entry, and therefore perforce unstreamed. And the smaller schools tend to be found in the poorest areas. We therefore calculated the partial correlation between streaming and attainment holding size of school constant. This reduces the correlation—but only from 0·46 to 0·33: it is still significant.

Backwardness and brightness

Let us now take a closer look at the average correlations with our measures of backwardness and brightness. As I have already mentioned, we find higher correlations with brightness, and this is true for both 'school' variables and 'social' variables: for the thirty-four school variables the average correlations with brightness and backwardness are 0·21 and 0·16 respectively; for the home and neighbourhood variables 0·29 and 0·26. When we look at the individual variables, we find only four having mean correlations greater than 0·4 with backwardness (cleanliness of home, 0·44; appearance and sociability, 0·42; verminous children, 0·42; and free meals, 0·42) while there are ten such with brightness. The four school variables having the strongest association with high scorers on the tests are: streaming, 0·47; attendance, 0·42; school size, 0·41; and percentage of children qualified for special schools, 0·41. The social variables over 0·4 emphasize again the *maternal care* factors that we have previously identified: verminous children, 0·50 ; mother working, 0·48 ; material needs inadequate, 0·48 ; free meals, 0·48 ; cleanliness of home, 0·46 ; and free clothing, 0·41.

It must be emphasized that these results have been obtained from an investigation of *schools* and not of individual children. We have found a correlation of 0·50, for example, between the percentage of verminous children in a school, and the percentage of high scorers on the tests given at four ages. Such results must be supported by parallel studies of individual children before one can begin to hazard a guess as to the underlying forces, and how they operate. Such studies are in hand, but I have as yet no results to report. Nevertheless, this association between brightness and environmental factors is a particularly important one. The potential profit if we can discover how to counteract such effects is very considerable. The evidence from the Manchester surveys, together with the work of Burt and Fraser, point to the virtual certainty that an adverse environment has its greatest educational effects on children of above average ability.*

Intelligence

Let us now turn to a comparison of the results from the tests of Intelligence with those from our tests of English and Arithmetic. The gross average correlations of all environmental variables with the three types of test show English and Intelligence (0·24 and 0·23) as slightly higher than Arithmetic (0·21). When we separate the social variables and the school variables, however, we find an interesting difference. For the home and neighbourhood variables the average r is 0·314 for Intelligence, 0·299 for English, and 0·262 for Arithmetic. The school variables put English clearly at the top (0·215) as against Intelligence, 0·190, and Arithmetic, 0·182.

* A recent interim report on a research by M. H. Maier on the academic achievement of adolescents, finds that " the high level scores . . . are positively correlated with socio-economic status and academic aptitude. The low level scores . . . have negative or close to zero correlations .." *E.T.S. Annual Report* 1963-64, p. 133.

These differences may seem relatively small, but it must be remembered that these are average correlations, and are based on a considerable number of single correlations. The least stable of these (IQ *v.* social) is derived from 162 separate coefficients, while English *v.* school variables is based on no fewer than 408.

We are now confronted with an interesting problem. Of the three kinds of test, why should IQ have the strongest association with the social variables? And why should the pattern be different for the school variables? I suggest that the crucial difference between the school variables and the home and neighbourhood variables lies in the fact that the latter are affected by, and affect, the *parents* of the children, while school variables are those which affect children only. In other words, I am emphasizing the heavier *genetic* element in the results of the intelligence tests. This is, at present, rather an unfashionable line to take, but in my view the evidence is inescapable. I do not intend to embark on a review of this evidence, but I may perhaps refer you to a recent survey by Erlenmeyer-Kimling and Jarvik (1963) [7] which summarizes fifty-two studies involving some 30,000 correlations. Figure 1 shows graphically the results of their analysis, which shows, as they point out, that " the *median* of the empirical correlations closely approaches the theoretical value predicted on the basis of genetic relationship alone. The average correlation between parent and child, as well as that between siblings (including dizygotic twins) is 0·50 . . . At the other end of the relationship scale, where monozygotic twins theoretically have 100 per cent genetic correlation, medians of the observed correlations in intellectual functioning are 0·87 for the twins brought up together, 0·75 for those brought up apart". The authors go on: " We do not imply that environment is without effect upon intellectual function ; the intellectual level is *not* unalterably fixed by the genetic constitution. Rather, its expression in the phenotype results from the patterns laid down by the genotype under given environmental conditions."

To return to our own results, I am arguing that much of the quality of the home and the neighbourhood is related to the parents' intellectual level. Adverse environments tend both to be produced by the incompetent and the incapable and also to

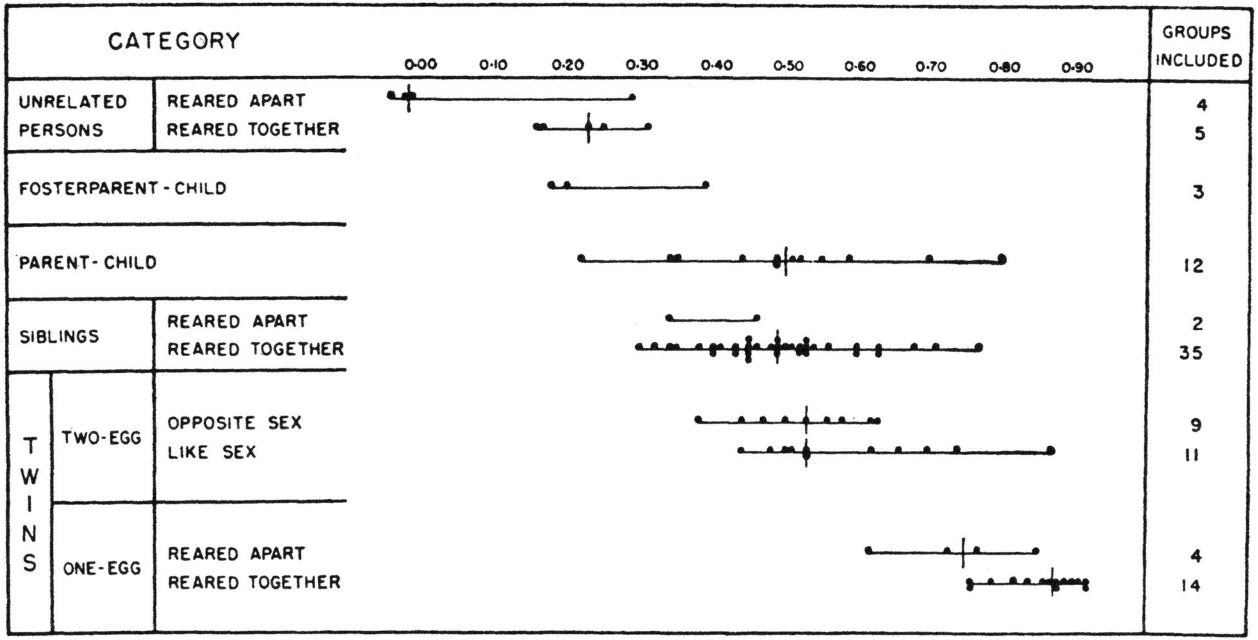

FIGURE 1

CORRELATION COEFFICIENTS FOR 'INTELLIGENCE' TEST SCORES FROM 52 STUDIES

Some studies reported data for more than one relationship category; some included more than one sample per category, giving a total of 99 groups. Over two-thirds of the correlation coefficients were derived from I.Q.'s, the remainder from special tests (for example, Primary Mental Abilities). Midparent-child correlation was used when available, otherwise mother-child correlation. Correlation coefficients obtained in each study are indicated by dark circles; medians are shown by vertical lines intersection the horizontal lines which represent the ranges.

attract them. And since there is a correlation of 0·5 between the intelligence of parents and that of their children, this produces a significant correlation between children's IQ and the social variables. A closer look at our average correlations supports this view. The social variables as a whole have a mean correlation of 0·28 with educational attainment. If, however, we break these down into 'home' variables and 'neighbourhood' variables, we find that the former have a mean *r* of 0·33 with attainment, the latter one of 0·18. The highest individual 'neighbourhood' correlation is 0·31 for Housing Standard. Eight of the 'home' variables are higher than this, and they range up to 0·48. Looking at the 'crime' variables, the criminal record of the family has an average correlation of 0·36 with the attainment tests, the criminal record of the neighbourhood 0·27, and that of the home address 0·05. Earlier in this paper I quoted Kemp's research, where a correlation of 0·73 between intelligence and attainment was reduced only to 0·62 when socio-economic status was partialled out. We get the same result on our own data. For example, the correlation between 10+ English and Intelligence is 0·82. If the effect of the social variables is held constant, this drops only to 0·80. With Arithmetic the fall is from 0·77 to 0·74.

In 1956 Ferguson [8] published an important paper "On transfer and the abilities of Man" which has received less attention than it deserved. In it he attempted to bring together learning theory and psychometrics, with a side-glance at the work of Piaget. He refers to Burnett's work on abilities of individuals living in relatively isolated communities. This "shows conclusively that the pattern of ability of children reared in relatively isolated outpost communities differs markedly from that of children reared in urban centres. In the isolated Newfoundland environment certain perceptive and motor abilities are developed to a high level, whereas verbal and reasoning abilities are less well developed. A retardation in abstract thinking and concept-formation seems to occur . . . Everything we know suggests that different environmental demands lead to the development of different ability patterns . . . The extensive body of literature on the abilities of individuals reared in cultures markedly different from our own in general supports this conclusion and adds substantial evidence for the role of learning in the formation of abilities " (p. 129). Ferguson suggests that differences in ability pattern resulting from differing environmental demands will show themselves not only in comparisons between indi-

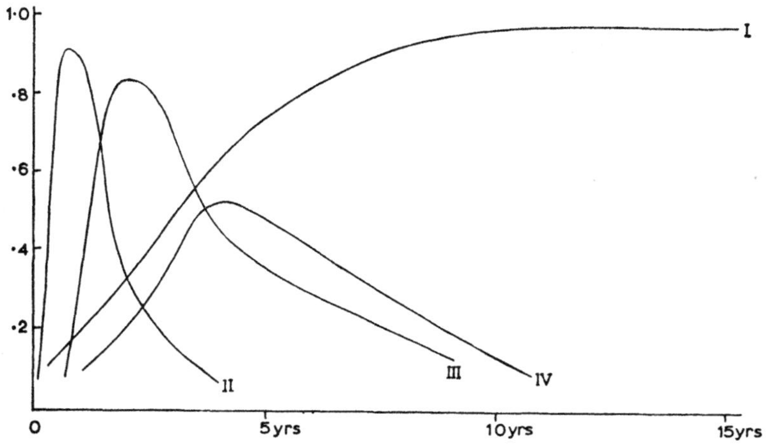

FIGURE 2

FACTOR LOADINGS DEVISED FROM AGE-LEVEL

Intercorrelations from the Californian growth study (Bayley, N., 1933, 1943, 1949 and 1951).

viduals reared in markedly different environments, but also in the same individual at different stages of growth, since environmental demands change radically as the child grows up. In other words, his hypothesis postulates different factor-patterns of ability at different ages. There is certainly some evidence of the truth of this. Figure 2 is based on the results from the Californian Growth Study, first reported by Bayley [1] in 1933, with additional data up to 1951. Bayley started testing the development and intelligence of a group of sixty-one infants within three days of birth, and continued testing them at stages up to the age of eighteen years. She provides a matrix of intercorrelation of the scores of the same individuals at ages ranging from 2 months to 210 months. In 1954 Hofstaetter[11] reported a factor analysis of this matrix, but since his centroid analysis was followed by rotation by hand, it was thought worth while to perform a new principle components analysis followed by a varimax rotation. Four major factors, as opposed to Hofstaetter's three, were found, and the loadings of these are plotted against age in the diagram. No clearer indication could be given of the change in factor-pattern with age. Factor I is clearly the one usually labelled ' intelligence ', but from birth up to at least the middle of the primary school this is supplemented by three other factors. I do not propose to embark on an attempt to ' label ' these factors, except to comment that, by inspection of the items of the Californian scale, Factor II (which finds its peak during the first year of life) is most probably a sensory-motor factor.

Our own survey provides test results at four different ages, and it is worth while seeing whether there is any variation in the pattern of correlation over the four years. Figure 3 shows average correlations of the three types of test for the home and neighbourhood variables and for the school variables separately. (It will be seen that all three tests were not included at every age.) Notice how the differentiation between the tests is greatest at 7+, and gets progressively less as the children get older. If we were able to extrapolate back into the infant school, no doubt the gaps would widen even more. And notice, too, the commanding position of the intelligence test for the home and neighbourhood variables.

I have some doubt as to whether the general upward trend of each single line on these graphs is really significant. It must be remembered that these correlations are between the test results of children who were ten years of age when the environmental variables were measured, so that the 10+ results and other variables are coincident in time. But the 7+ results are those of these same children three years ago, the 8+ two years ago, and so on. It would not be surprising therefore, if these correlations have been subject to some degree of shrinkage. If so, the possibility exists that the level of correlation may *fall* with age. A comparison of our primary school results with those from secondary schools in 1957, using pupils of 14+, certainly suggests that this is so. The correlations of attainment with environmental variables all tend to be higher at 10+ than at 14+. Two of the social variables were identical in the two surveys: percentage of verminous children, and percentage in receipt of free shoes and clothing. The average correlations of the former with attainment were 0·483 at 10+, 0·383 at 14+ ; for the latter the figures are 0·237 and 0·173. The fall from 10+ to 14+ is apparent for all three types of test, with the change for arithmetic being rather

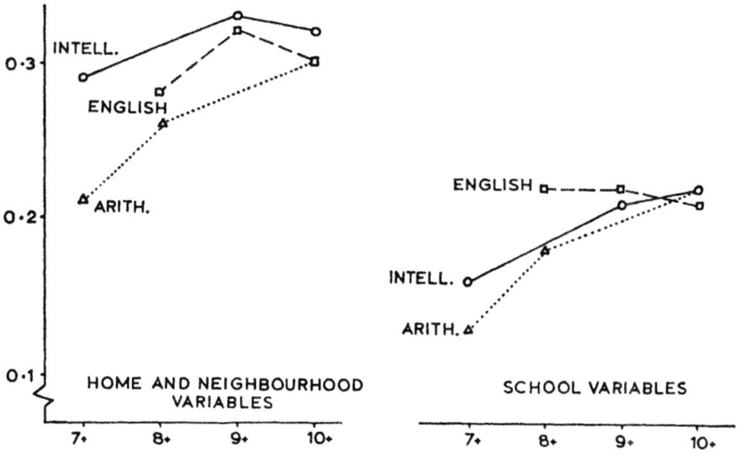

FIGURE 3

MEAN CORRELATIONS

greater than for English, the smallest change being with the intelligence test.

It seems, then, that not only do we find different patterns of ability at different age-levels, but also that the impact of environmental factors on attainment gets progressively weaker as we go up the age-range. There are other pieces of evidence which support this age-trend. Furneaux,[10] in his book *The Chosen Few* (1961), comments on the fact that " occupational group membership acts as a very important determinant of academic history throughout the stages of education up to that of entry to the sixth form ", but then goes on: " The proportion of those wishing to have a university education who are actually able to apply is much the same for pupils in all occupational groups ", and again: " Among pupils who have already reached the upper-sixth form, differences of home background are associated only to a very small degree with the strength of the desire for a university education." This analysis of sixth formers receives strong support from the evidence provided by the Robbins Committee, who comment (App. I, p. 46): " The proportion of working-class children who stay on to the age when A-level is normally attempted is smaller than the proportion of middle-class children who actually achieve two passes. But these working-class children who do stay on are on average as successful as their counterparts in other social groups." The Committee present data connecting 11+ results with A-level performance, classifying pupils into top, middle and bottom thirds on 11+ results. They find: " Within each ability group at 11+, there is no significant difference in performance between children from the different classes who stay on ". Table I presents the Robbins data from the relevant table of the Report, and from this it is clear that differences of social class have ceased to be effective determinants of achievement at this level and at this age.

From the evidence so far discussed, it seems to be likely: *first,* that the influence of environmental factors on educational attainment is greatest at the youngest ages, and gets progressively less influential as the children get older ; *second,* that as far as social class is concerned—a very crude measure of environmental differences—its effect seems to disappear by the age of seventeen or eighteen* ; *third,* that factors in the home and neighbourhood, and particularly those associated with maternal care and material needs, are much more powerful determinants of educational achievement than are factors within the walls of the school itself ; *fourth,* that the stronger association between the intelligence test results and

* There is a suggestion from the USA that with college students " economic advantage is by no means positively related to academic achievement, and, in fact, that the relationship which might be expected from the term ' advantage ' is actually reversed ". (Crawford, 1929.) [6]

the 'home' variables suggest that their primacy of effect might be due largely to genetic factors; and *fifth*, that adverse forces in the environment have their greatest effect on the more able children.

The question now arises, what can we do to counteract the effects of poor environment? The prognosis is bleak, since it seems more than likely that the greatest harm to the child occurs before ever he reaches school at five years of age, and that any efforts the school might make are rather in the nature of shutting the stable door after the horse has bolted.

TABLE I

PERCENTAGE OF SCHOOL LEAVERS AGED 18 OR MORE WHO HAVE AT LEAST 2 A-LEVELS

(From Table 7, p. 45, Appendix I of the Robbins Report)

	11+ Grading		
Father's Occupation	Upper third	Middle third	Lower third
Professional and managerial	79	63	43
Clerical	74	56	58
Skilled manual	77	59	51
Semi- and un-skilled	81	58	53

But this may be too pessimistic a view, and it would certainly be premature to conclude that ameliorative action on the part of teachers and local authorities is unlikely to have much effect. What such action should be, however, and what chances it has of success, cannot be decided until we know something about causality. So far we have been dealing with correlations, with measures of association. The leap from these to causal factors is a hazardous and difficult one. Piaget [16] has charted certain stages in the intellectual development of the child and has demonstrated the interaction between the child's abilities and the environment's opportunities. As he says: "Life is a continuous creation of increasingly complex forms and a progressive adaptation of these forms to the environment" (Piaget 1936, p. 3).[16] There is much evidence from both animals and from children that environmental deprivation not only slows down development, but may permanently lower the level of later performance. These intellectual and logical schemata of Piaget may have their counterpart in the effective and creative life of children, and particularly of pre-school children. The years before five are notoriously crucial for the development of mental health: they may be equally so for educational health. It is perhaps unnecessary to see the required causal links through Freudian spectacles. For my part I would prefer to go back to McDougall and suggest that at least part of the system of causality lies in the emergence of the self-regarding sentiment in the pre-school child. This, nourished in the home, is the architect of the child's attitude to authority, and structures his decisions as to which environmental opportunities he accepts and which he rejects. I have no time to do more than to indicate a possible line of approach here, but it is one which, in my view, demands further exploration. Psychologists and sociologists have often interested themselves in the suburban phenomenon of keeping up with the Joneses: it is time they took a more intensive look at the parallel phenomenon in the lower socio-economic echelons, that of keeping down with the Smiths.

If part of the system of causality is revealed along such lines, then it follows that the best hope of ameliorative action lies not so much in improvements in the physical environment of the child's home, his neighbourhood and his school *—necessary though these are from other points of view—not in organizational changes within the school itself, but rather in a reorientation of our training of teachers. They must not only be made aware of the nature of the adverse forces with which they are faced, but they must be expected to engage in positive action with parents as well as children. It would be wildly unrealistic to suggest that all teachers, and primary school teachers in particular, should be trained as social workers as well as educators, but the careful selection of a proportion of teachers for specialist training for general liaison work between school and home is a perfectly feasible proposition. Movement in this direction has already begun, but it needs rapid acceleration if any sensible impact is to be made on the

* And, of course, as has been emphasized by other contributors, a considerable increase in the provision of nursery schools in the worst areas.

problem, and if we hope to rescue at least a proportion of the large number of potentially able children who, at present, sink down under the weight of so many adverse conditions.

DISCUSSION

A questioner asked the lecturer to amplify his explanation of the correlations between home variables and intelligence tests, and their connection with the argument he later developed regarding compensating factors in the school. PROFESSOR WISEMAN replied that this was an additional and complementary mechanism ; he believed that the argument he used of compensation by the teachers in the schools in the worst areas was one which applied much more to the secondary than to the primary school stage. He thought that there was a difference here, and (though it was early yet, and he would have liked to have had more information and analysis of the Manchester data) that probably both these worked together in a complementary way in the primary school, and that the compensatory principle was stronger in the secondary school.

REFERENCES

1. BAYLEY, N. 1933. Mental growth during the first three years: a developmental study of 61 children by repeated tests. *Genet. Psychol. Monog.* **14**, 1.
2. BAYLEY, N. 1943. Mental growth during the first three years. In *Child Behaviour and Development.* (Ed. R. G., Barker, J. S. Kounin and H. F. Wright). New York. McGraw-Hill.
3. BAYLEY, N. 1949. Consistency and variability in the growth of intelligence from birth to 18 years. *J. Genet. Psychol.* **75**, 165-196.
4. BAYLEY, N. 1951. Development and maturation. In *Theoretical Foundation of Psychology.* (Ed. H. Helson). New York. Van Nostrand.
5. BURT, C. 1943. Ability and income. *Brit. J. educ. Psychol.* **13**, 83-98.
6. CRAWFORD, A. B. 1929. *Incentives to Study.* New Haven, Yale University Press.
7. ERLENMEYER-KIMLING, L. and JARVIK, L. F. 1963. Genetics and intelligence: a review. *Science* **142**, No. 3598.
8. FERGUSON, G. A. 1956. On transfer and the abilities of Man. *Canad. J. Psychol.* **8**, 121-131.

9. FRASER, E. D. 1959. *Home Environment and the School.* London. University of London Press.
10. FURNEAUX, W. D. 1961. *The Chosen Few.* London. Oxford University Press.
11. HOFSTAETTER, P. R. 1954. The changing composition of 'intelligence': a study in T-technique. *J. Genet. Psychol.* **85**, 159-164.
12. KEMP, L. C. D. 1955. Environmental and other characteristics determining attainments in primary schools. *Brit. J. educ. Psychol.* **25**, 67-77.
13. MAXWELL, J. 1953. *Social Implications of the 1947 Scottish Mental Survey.* London. University of London Press.
14. MINISTRY OF EDUCATION. 1963. *Higher Education* (The Robbins Report). App. I. London. H.M.S.O.
15. MOLLENKOPF, W. G. 1956. A study of secondary school characteristics determining attainment. *Educ. Test. Service Res. Bull.* **56**, No. 6.
16. PIAGET, J. 1936. *The Origins of Intelligence in Children.* New York. Int. Univ. Press.
17. WISEMAN, S. 1964. *Education and Environment.* Manchester. Manchester University Press.

THE LIMITS OF PREDICTION

JAMES DREVER
Department of Psychology, University of Edinburgh

WERE I to talk about the circumstance which seems to me more than any other to limit prediction in Higher Education—both the prediction of individual success and the estimate of total numbers capable of a particular level of academic work—I should discuss, not the intelligence of candidates, but the foibles of examiners. Our forecasts are validated against a criterion which has been shown again and again to be unreliable, yet each of us seems able to persuade himself that it is other examiners who go astray, and in general that with care and patience we can make the present system work well enough. This view is not unreasonable when we have in mind the random lapses of attention and changes of mood to which we are all subject—what I have called the 'noise' in the system [2]—but it is not true of adaptation. Human beings are incredibly adaptable to slow consistent changes of any kind. As a result what they respond to as neutral or normal or average, within quite wide limits, is not anchored in the outside world, but varies with their own past experience, especially their recent past experience. This can produce 'drift', a steady change in standards over time. In consequence a bad selection procedure will frequently seem less bad than it is, and a good one less good: while the estimate of total numbers always has to protect itself by laying down an unfulfilled condition, namely that assessment should remain constant. There are ways of solving this problem, some laborious, some technical, but these are not in common use; so I must begin with the warning that any statistical or genetic study taking performance in current academic examinations as a datum is sure to run into trouble. Even administrative decisions on such a basis are dangerous: scientific conclusions cannot be drawn.

But the auspices under which we are met here make inappropriate a further pursuit of this line of argument at this stage. What I propose to do is illustrate, by means of two case histories, some of the points made by others. Although there are lessons to be drawn from these in the prediction of individual success and failure, my main concern is with the much bigger problem of detecting the presence in the population at large of such endowment as would make higher education possible at all. In particular, I hope to bring out the essentially historical and individual nature of many of the variables we are trying to assess.

My cases are two young ladies, Alice and Olive, both aged twenty at the time of the investigation. I should explain that it has been the custom in Edinburgh from time to time, since 1935, to subject the big first-year class in Psychology to various intelligence tests. Over the years about five thousand students have produced scores of one sort or another. The test with the longest period of use is one constructed by Sir Cyril Burt for Sixth-formers: Group Test 33. It is a verbal test and gives a modest correlation with academic performance. Alice was our top-scorer, and in fact made full marks: Olive was our lowest by a considerable margin. The norms for the test are not very satisfactory so far as the general population is concerned, but Olive was slightly below the mean on these norms. This difference was a real one and was confirmed by subsequent performance in other tests. Alice was not quite so good with non-verbal material but she made consistently high scores on every test we used. On the parallel version of the test she first took she was only two short of a possible. Olive remained around the mean for the general population where norms were available, and right outside any student distribution that I have seen.

Both graduated M.A. Ordinary, and trained as teachers. Alice married a year later, and I daresay Olive too is married now. She was a pleasant-looking, and, in her way, a friendly girl.

Any surprise that you may feel at the disparity of apparent endowment and similarity of achievement may easily be dispelled by a few biographical details. Alice was the daughter of two teachers, an only child who came to them relatively late in life. Thus she was exposed early to a wide vocabulary, and did not have to be good or clever to gain affection ; it was enough for her parents that she was there. So she grew up secure, literate, wide-ranging in her interests, but rather easy-going. What has been called her need for achievement hardly existed.

Olive, on the other hand, was one of five. There were three brothers, two older than herself, and a younger sister. Her father was a small farmer in the North-east of Scotland, and her mother also came from a farming family. They were Free Presbyterians, that is they belonged to a sect which regards the ordinary Scottish presbyterian as worldly and frivolous. For some reason Olive was regarded as the clever one of the family, and their ambition was for her to become a teacher, preferably a graduate teacher. We hear a great deal nowadays about the low esteem in which teaching is held, but in the remoter country districts of Scotland it is still regarded as the height of feminine ambition. A clever boy may become a doctor or a minister, but for a girl status is to be found in front of the blackboard. So Olive came under pressure quite early, and yet you must not think of her as driven into academic pursuits by ambitious parents. So long as she could remember, the choice and ambition were hers too. She was physically robust, emotionally stable, and not inclined to worldly pleasures. She worked prodigiously, failed quite often, but in the end, though it took her a long time, she attained her goal.

So you see there is no real problem: our two cases have an almost copybook quality. We have, do we not, a clever, idle girl, and a dim industrious one, so in the end they achieve much the same? Well, of course, that may be the answer ; but let us go on now and take a look at some more evidence.

First of all let us consider rather more closely their academic performance. They wrote, as you might expect, very different kinds of papers. Alice was copious, with an immense vocabulary, a tendency to wander from the point, and some liability to error. She gave the impression that she did not know her material very well, and was sometimes trying to talk herself out of trouble. Nevertheless she received quite good marks in all subjects, and passed her degree examinations at the first attempt. Olive produced short meagre answers, suggestive of rote learning. She made few mistakes and her sins were of omission. As I have said, she failed frequently, and in fact took six years to complete her degree. Nowadays she would have been sent down at the end of her first year.

The picture still seems quite consistent with the obvious explanation, but there is something about the qualitative differences I have just pointed out which suggests another line of argument. The question is whether in fact these two girls were innately so different from one another as appearances seem to indicate. Since I am more of an experimental than an educational psychologist, I must leave human beings for a little and turn to rats.

Some of you will remember the interesting case of Tryon's [6] maze-learning strain. These rats were selectively bred for many generations to be good at running mazes. In the end the strain became so good at this that even its slowest members were better than the best unselected ones. At the time the difference was regarded as an intellectual one, if I may so use the term, and a Tryon rat was thought to be a clever rat. Subsequent investigations using other tasks showed that this was not so at all. The Tryon rats were greedy, active, get-up-and-go rats, but no cleverer than the others. They bustled about their mazes with exceptional zeal, and so gave the impression of being what in fact they were not. I mention this incident to call attention to the risks attendant on the inference from behaviour to some particular innate characteristic.

Still among the rats but closer to our own problem, there is an interesting early study by Tolman,[5] also of maze-learning. He used a sectional maze in which the pathways could be modified. Two groups of rats learned a route to the food-box which involved a considerable detour. One group was normally hungry, the other very hungry indeed. When both had learned the long route a shorter one was opened. The normally hungry rats switched quickly to the new way, even though they had taken the other over and over again. The very hungry rats, by contrast, kept to the now unnecessary detour. Somehow excessive motivation had made them rigid and unable to exploit the alternative possibility. As Tolman put it, they had learned a strip map in which only the details along the way were remembered. The overall pattern of the maze was not apparent to them and so their hunger made them less intelligent.

Now this is not an isolated finding: it has been confirmed repeatedly. Bruner and his associates,[1] for example, found that if two groups of rats were trained to make a sequence of turns, LRLR, and then the starting point were changed so that the required pattern became RLRL, the moderately motivated group, after a period of puzzlement, were able to change quite quickly. The highly motivated group, on the other hand, though they learned the new starting point, could only follow it with the now inappropriate LRLR. " It would seem then," says Bruner, " that under conditions of high drive, if a path to a goal has been learned, it is learned, so to speak, as ' *this* path to *this* goal ' and is not coded or acquired as an example of a more generic pattern, ' this *kind* of path to this *kind* of goal '. In consequence, when a new situation arises, the driven creature does not have a generic coding system that permits him to go beyond it ' insightfully '. It is as if one of the students of geometry in Wertheimer's study (1945) had learned to do the operations necessary for solving the area of *this* parallelogram but had not generalized the knowledge into a coding system for handling parallelograms of slightly different size, shape, or position."

Other species exhibit the same phenomenon. Monkeys were shown by Harlow[3] to acquire generic concepts most easily when the reward was minimal. If the outcome became too important the learning became specific. Human beings similarly have been shown in a wide variety of circumstances to suffer a decline in flexibility and originality under stress. Necessity may not be the mother of invention after all.

Perhaps I should call attention to the fact that the drives which seem to upset the more complex kinds of learning are always extrinsic to the learning process itself. Too much hunger, thirst, or anxiety, can be damaging, but I doubt whether intense curiosity would be.

You may wonder what all this has to do with intelligence. After all, these effects of motive and stress are transient, while intelligence is assumed to be a relatively enduring characteristic. Perhaps this is so, at least by the time we come to measure it, but I should defend the relevance of the experiments I have just cited by reminding you, as did Professor Vernon, of a very important distinction drawn by Hebb in 1949.[4] Using evidence from the effects of brain injury occurring early and later in life he claimed that " the word ' intelligence ' has two valuable meanings. One (A) is an innate potential, the capacity for development, a fully innate property that amounts to the possession of a good brain and a good neural metabolism. The second (B) is the functioning of a brain in which development has already gone on, determining an *average level of performance or comprehension* by the partly grown or mature person. Neither, of course, is observed directly ; but intelligence B, a hypothetical level of development of brain function, is a much more direct inference from behaviour than intelligence A, the original potential."

Hebb went on to point out, " Most of the disagreement in recent years over the nature of ' intelligence ' concerns the relation of A, innate potential, to B, the estimated level of functioning at maturity. If A determines B fully, intelligence is a matter of heredity and maturation only ; the IQ is not dependent on experience. But if intelligence A is only *one* of the conditions of intelligence B, not the sole determinant, what then ? . . .

" The dispute in the current literature has arisen, I believe, partly because of the double reference of the term ' intelligence ', and partly because it has not been realized that if the effects of early experience are more or less generalized and permanent, one can concede a major effect of experience on the IQ and still leave the IQ its constancy and validity as an index of future performance ". This last is the important point for our present discussion. It would seem that the grand strategy of our thinking develops out of our early experience to an extent not yet widely recognized. Once it has developed, however, it is as basic and stable a component in our make-up as any that arises entirely from genetic factors.

We do not know very much at present about the many and subtle influences which must enter into the transition from intelligence A to intelligence B. Clearly learning is central. That is to say, so long as we think of intelligence as the variable which is measured by intelligence tests then it is partly true to say that we learn to be intelligent, though limits are set by heredity. This, of course, is just another way of saying that we can learn to be stupid. It would seem to follow that the kind of excessive motivation which produces a transient impairment in the learning of an adult organism may do permanent damage if it is at all prevalent at an earlier stage when basic cognitive strategies are being built up.

Let us return to Alice and Olive now, and take a second look at their thinking in the light of these considerations. You remember the difference between them. Faced with a problem, Alice would generate possible solutions with great freedom, showing flexibility and resourcefulness. In matching these solutions to the requirements of the problem she was on the whole less impressive. Where the matching was easy, as in the clear-cut answers to test items, she did extremely well, but in circumstances where information and judgement were important she showed some deficiencies. Olive, on the other hand, seemed to suffer from a sort of cognitive constipation, if you forgive the term, and in the task of generating possible solutions she could produce very little. She was unoriginal, and, where it might help, she relied on rote learning. On the other hand, in the matching phase of the operation, where possible solutions were compared with the requirements of the problem, Olive did better with what she had in the sense that proportionally as well as absolutely she made fewer mistakes. Alice was adventurous, original, and her errors did not worry her. Olive was timid, careful, and persistent. You notice how I am forced to use adjectives which are not restricted in their application to merely cognitive operations. This is as it should be. If the style is the man, so much more is his whole way of intellectual life.

You will also have noticed, I hope, how closely the two ways of intellectual life that I have chosen for comparison resemble the behaviour of Tolman's rats and Harlow's monkeys at different levels of motivation. Perhaps by this time you are becoming uneasily aware of a possible alternative to the obvious explanation for the unequal gifts and similar achievements of our two cases. This was to the effect that Alice did only moderate academic work in spite of her high intelligence, because of low motivation. In plain terms she was spoilt and lazy. Olive, on the other hand, graduated eventually in spite of her low intelligence, because of high motivation. What I have tried to do is suggest that there are some grounds for supposing that the intelligence as well as the academic performance has been subject to motivational influences, and that here these have been in precisely the opposite direction. If getting the right answer had been made too important for Alice at an early age, we might never have had the rapid and confident thinking which gave her such high test scores ; while Olive, in a less bleak and exacting context, might have shown qualities of mind which now she does not have. All this is surmise, of course, but so is the plain tale with which we started. My varnished one in fact can offer more strictly experimental evidence in its support. We do not have to choose, since both can be true.

Now at length we are in a position to consider the implications of this kind of evidence for the problem of predicting in the long run numbers in higher education. They would seem to me to be far-reaching. As I have said, the factors which determine the transition from intelligence as inherited to intelligence as measured are largely unknown to us. I have directed your attention to one such factor only ; there may be many. Imagination and experiment have begun to probe the possibilities. Froebel, Montessori, and Piaget, have made their different kinds of contribution. But if we find, when more is known, as I believe we shall find, that much can be done to nurture intelligence as well as train or measure it at a later stage, then our educational budgeting must bear this in mind. Twelve per cent of a population, subjected to the largely random interplay of influence prevalent in the environment of young children to-day are thought capable of profiting by higher education as we know it. What the figure will be when the nurture of intelligence B is more fully understood cannot now be determined. It is sure to be greater, and may be much greater.

This brings me back to the point at which I began. Changes when they come, will come slowly; unless we are on our guard, the system of higher education will adapt to them, without realizing that they have occurred. We may see a gradual rise in academic standards, the consequence of which would be to exclude indefinitely some 88 per cent of an age group. I hope I have said enough to show that, if this does happen—and the danger is a real one—it cannot be justified by the claim that intelligence, in the sense that matters, is innate, and can be expected to remain constant in a population from year to year and from decade to decade.

REFERENCES

1. Bruner, J. S. 1957. Going beyond the information given. In *Contemporary Approaches to Cognition.* Cambridge, Mass. Harvard University Press, p. 41.
2. Drever, J. 1965. Need, choice, and supply in Higher Education. *Advan. Sci., Lond.* **22**, 95, 29.
3. Harlow, H. F. 1949. The formation of learning sets. *Psychol. Rev.* **56**, 51.
4. Hebb, D. O. 1949. *The Organization of Behavior.* New York. Wiley.
5. Tolman, E. C. 1938. Cognitive maps in rats and men. *Psychol. Rev.* **45**, 1.
6. Tryon, R. C. 1940. Genetic differences in maze-learning ability in rats. *Thirty-ninth Yb. Nat. Soc. Stud. Educ.* 111.

SELECTION AND THE PROBLEM OF CONFORMITY

LIAM HUDSON
Research Centre, King's College, Cambridge

AN assumption widely held amongst teachers and psychologists, throughout the educational systems of all countries, is that their pupils are reasonably consistent. It is assumed that the boy who excels at the age of ten or eleven will still be doing well a decade later—that he will have gained outstanding 'O' Level and 'A' Level results, and perhaps a university scholarship too, and that he is destined to take a First Class degree. Everyone admits exceptions—the 'late starters', and the precocious children who begin brilliantly but fail to fulfil their early promise. What is not clear, however, is how numerous these exceptions may be. There is little evidence of a searching nature that bears on this point, and experts are still free to disagree. Some argue that the level of consistency in intellectual performance is high from one age level to another. Others counter—and for a variety of reasons—that such consistency in children is less real than apparent.

No attempt will be made in this paper to resolve this dispute in its general form. I shall, however, discuss one particular corner of it. I wish to examine the relation of success *within* the school and University system to success in the world at large; to review the evidence relating school marks and degree classes on the one hand, to intellectual achievement amongst adults on the other. And on the basis of such empirical evidence, I shall draw some morals about practices now current in university selection.

Some eight years ago, I carried out a small study of eminent scientists. Specifically, I examined the classes gained in Tripos and Final Honours Schools by Fellows of the Royal Society and by members of Oxford and Cambridge holding the degree of Doctor of Science. (The samples were restricted to those who had taken their first degree during the period 1920-39). I was surprised to find that a large proportion of such scientists had performed indifferently at university ; at some time in their university careers quite a large number had gained Seconds, some Lower Seconds, and a few had gained Thirds or even Fourths. In fact, the classes of Degree gained by Fellows of the Royal Society or Doctors of Science did not seem to differ significantly—at Cambridge, at least—from those gained by contemporaries of the same age and sex, who took the same subject in the same year, and went into research at the same time, but did not become Fellows of the Royal Society or Doctors of Science. In the Cambridge sample, for example, 23 per cent of the FRSs gained a Second or Third Class in their final degrees, as compared with 21 per cent in the control group; 43 per cent of the DScs gained Seconds or Thirds, whereas only 31 per cent of the controls did so. Among research workers, in other words, there seemed no positive relation between degree class and scientific accomplishment.[3]

I looked at other groups, too ; at Cabinet Ministers, for example, comparing them with non-Cabinet Ministers, and with ordinary back-bench MPs. I looked also at High Court Judges and compared them with County Court Judges. In both cases, there was evidence of some slight relation between eminence and degree class, but it was far from clear-cut, and there were many striking exceptions. Two of the most intellectually distinguished of our High Court Judges, for instance, gained, respectively, two Lower Seconds, and a Lower Second and a Third, as Cambridge undergraduates. Of High Court Judges, 54 per cent had gained Seconds or worse ; 24 per cent had taken Thirds, Fourths or Ordinary degrees. Only 10 per cent of County Court Judges had taken Firsts. There were similar equally pointed anomalies among Cabinet Ministers. Sixty-six per cent of Ministers holding Cabinet rank during the period 1945-59 gained Seconds, Thirds or Fourths at Oxford or Cambridge ; and the equivalent figures for non-Cabinet Ministers and back-benchers were 87 per cent and 85 per cent respectively. Those generally reputed to have the greatest intellectual ability (or the greatest political acumen) sometimes had university careers which we would now regard as calamitous.[4]

Such findings may seem a little hard to accept. Nevertheless, they are in precise agreement with the results of much larger and more distinguished pieces of research conducted in the United States. MacKinnon, for example, has studied outstanding mathematicians, scientists, engineers, architects, and writers. One of his most interesting findings was that at school and at College these men and women were, to use the American idiom, 'B' or often 'C' students—that is, only a little better than the average run.[7] However, MacKinnon does remark of those students who were later to become great figures in science or architecture or literature, that they sometimes showed their ability when a special interest was aroused. If a particular subject took their fancy, they worked hard and gained a good mark; for the rest, however, they seemed content to do little work, or none at all.

Other American psychologists have attempted to predict the abilities of young research scientists on the basis of their examination results; again findings have been largely negative ones.[2] It simply is not a fact that we can use school marks or degree classes to predict who will do well in mature intellectual work and who will not. The relation between success within the academic sphere and other kinds of intellectual success seems relatively slight.

It seems that what holds true for school marks and university degrees applies also to the results of psychological tests. Though both school examinations and intelligence tests differentiate, in a broad way, between the bright and the dull, they seem not to differentiate significantly between those intelligent people who realize their intellectual potentialities in some concrete form and those intellectual people who do not. We may use psychological tests to predict, at least moderately well, the performance of school children in school examinations—as has been demonstrated, for example, in the eleven-plus examination.[9] This relation between test scores and marks also holds good to some extent for undergraduates. It is normally assumed, for example, that intelligence test scores will correlate to the extent of $+0{\cdot}5$ with marks gained in multiple choice examinations—that is, they will account for a quarter of the variation in those examinations.

Most evidence suggests that the same holds true in this country, although correlations are usually lower. My own findings, based on fifteen-year-old schoolboys who later win Open Scholarships and take First Class degrees at Oxford and Cambridge, suggest that at university this relation between test scores and academic results becomes very tenuous indeed. For example, 24 per cent of future winners of Open Scholarships and Exhibitions fell within the bottom 30 per cent of my sample in IQ. Future Open Scholars were distinguished not by their test scores, but by their tendency to work hard, and by the breadth of their interests outside the curriculum.[5]

Many individual cases illustrate this point ; two, perhaps, will serve. The first is a boy who, at the age of sixteen, was judged by his teachers to be one of the school's best prospects in the physical sciences. He was a good physicist, was gifted musically, and, in general, was a lively and charming member of the school community. He later gained an Open Scholarship to Cambridge, and recently took a First in Physics. Yet his intelligence quotient was lower than that of some 80 per cent of his class-mates, some of whom left school with no 'A' levels at all.

The second case concerns a young mathematician. At fifteen, his intelligence quotient was just a little above the average of his form. There was nothing, however, about the profile of his test results to suggest the brilliant future which his teachers foretold. He too won an Open Scholarship, took Part III of the Mathematical Tripos in three years, and also won the top Mathematics prize. In academic terms, at least, he is clearly one of the ablest young mathematicians of his age in the country. The tests I used were the best then available ; they were given under good conditions ; and there is no question that the boys concentrated upon them at least reasonably hard. Moreover, they were not exceptions. Boys who later won Open Scholarships at Oxford and Cambridge differ only very slightly in their mental test scores from class-mates who go there as Commoners, who go to other universities, or who leave school and go to no university at all. In other words, it seems that, once they have reached the Sixth Form, the abilities of boys to do conventional mental tests are not closely related to their subsequent achievement—even in examinations, not to mention later life.

This finding, again, is in accord with the American research on eminent men. Both Roe [8] and MacKinnon [7] agree that men and women of the highest intellectual distinction are not differentiated from their less successful contemporaries by their mental test scores. On the strength of this, MacKinnon goes on to argue that above a certain level, somewhere in the region of IQ 115-125, conventional intelligence has little bearing on subsequent intellectual achievement. A similar interpretation sits neatly upon the findings of my own which I have just described.

In the United States, many senior psychologists concerned with university selection seem now to accept this predictive failure of psychological tests as given, and—at the research level at least—to be looking elsewhere for an accurate basis of selection. In particular, one finds there a marked interest in the obsessive quality of most productive intellectuals' lives. And in America, where the search for scientific talent is a serious matter, this capacity for obsessive, all-absorbing interest in a particular topic is now the focus of the keenest attention. One also finds close attention paid to a quality which most English teachers view with distaste—a student's *lack* of intellectual discipline. MacKinnon, and also Professor Bloom,[1] have evidence to suggest not merely that original thinkers lack intellectual discipline as students, but that this very lack of discipline, their erraticness, is an important prognostic sign. On this argument, the original thinker of the future is the student who works when he is interested and is prone to idle when he is not.

I now wish to point some morals about university selection. university selection, especially in institutions like Oxford and Cambridge, is increasingly a matter of open competition for conventional academic honours. Increasingly, the criterion for admission is that of three good results in the GCE 'A' level examination ; and as we are becoming more democratic in our patterns of recruitment, as we get more applications from schools which in the past would not have sent boys to Oxford or Cambridge, so the pace is sharpening. Until quite recently, it was possible to gain entrance to Oxford or Cambridge on the strength of one's family connections, as Charles Darwin did. As recently as the early 1950s, it was possible to be offered a Cambridge place on the strength of one's accomplishment on the athletics field, plus two ' A ' levels of any quality at all. This is no longer so. Competition is increasingly severe ; and the criteria, despite the retention of Scholarship examinations, more and more restricted. Every year there is less space in the University entrance system for young men and young women who seem to have intellectual potentialities beyond their demonstrable academic accomplishment.

There would seem to be great dangers in such a situation. First, there is the question of recruitment. A central aim of our universities is, presumably, to give an intellectual training to those young men and women who are most likely to be intellectually productive as adults. Yet, if this is so, we are admitting many whom we ought to fail, and failing many we should admit. In other words, if we may rely at all on empirical evidence, our selection is at fault. Secondly, there is the question of failure and its effects on the majority who are not admitted, either to the University of their first choice, or to any University at all. If the chief criterion of intellectual merit is that of ' O ' level and ' A ' level results, and a particular child has poor ' O ' levels and ' A ' levels, we, as teachers or selectors, are bound unintentionally to undermine whatever self-confidence he may possess. Thus the present examination system seems doubly wasteful: it fails to select many of the candidates it is designed to select, and it may also have grave ill effects on talented individuals whom it fails. Thirdly, there is the question of conformity. The keener the competition and the more clearly defined the criteria of success, the greater the influence of our examination system on the intellectual standards of the children whose futures depend upon it. In other words, the greater the academic pressure, the more nearly our educational system comes to resemble a system of indoctrination.

One is tempted to criticize any educational system which conditions children to find the right answer—the answer, that is, which the *examiner* defines as right. But in the light of recent American evidence, there seems a special case for criticizing systems which not merely demand excellence, in strictly defined academic terms, but which demand it all round. For it seems that it is precisely the demand for all-round excellence, for good 'A' level results not in one subject but in three, which is an especially dubious feature of the university selection system now evolving. This evidence—the results of MacKinnon, Roe and Bloom—suggests that the ability to channel one's interests, even obsessively, may be a condition for producing original work. It may be, in other words, that the ability to turn one's hand to any task is not necessarily an unalloyed advantage. Instead of describing such people as 'brilliant all-rounders', perhaps we should begin to view them instead as 'intellectually labile', or even as 'intellectually promiscuous'.

When tests and examinations are given to children (or to adults) it is normally assumed that each individual will try hard, that he will do his best. Yet it may be, in the cases of the inventive and original especially, that certain individuals focus their minds closely only on topics which they find of absorbing interest. Thus a large number of men and women capable of both originality and devotion to their mature intellectual work will perform poorly in tests and examinations designed to tap their 'knowledge', their 'intelligence' or, for that matter, their 'creativeness'. If this is so, then one can only hope to measure such individuals' capabilities by setting them problems *within* their sphere of special interest. The only way in which we can judge the abilities of a boy who is interested solely in the construction of logical computers is to judge how well his logical computers compute.

Yet if we allow that such specificity of interest may exist (and we can scarcely deny it), we are forced to make some revealing admissions. We must envisage a spectrum of individuals, ranging from those who can apply their full energy to any task to those who can apply themselves only when their special interests are aroused. Traditionally, teachers and psychologists are inclined to view this second group as handicapped; and such boys do stand at a practical disadvantage in that they will fail tests and examinations which their more amenable contemporaries pass. Yet in setting such children examinations we may be penalizing precisely those qualities of independence, dedication and rapacious interest which we should hope to foster.[6]

Clearly, this train of thought should not be allowed to discredit our present system of examinations and mental tests in its entirety. Nevertheless, it illuminates a grave weakness of which many mental testers and teachers are guilty alike. We are prone to use tests and examinations as simple, global criteria of an individual's intellectual calibre. Moreover, we base our expectations of him upon our assessments of his test and examination results. This, it could be argued, is poor psychology and poor teaching. Doubtless, individuals do differ in their native endowment: it may well be that, however well we are taught, some of us will never master circuit diagrams, or the proper use of the semi-colon. What I do wish to suggest, though, is that we should not make assumptions about the limits of a child's potentialities until we have exhausted every conceivable means of eliciting them. From the practical point of view of the university selector, we face, moreover, a paradox. If we set out to make university entrance (or indeed any form of intellectual advantage) a matter of open, democratic competition, we achieve not a system in which children are free to develop their intellectual interests and potentialities, but quite the reverse—a system in which intellectual docility and conformity are the highest virtues.

Granted that this danger exists, what is the practical remedy? Will it be avoided, for example, if university places are provided for all who wish to occupy them? The briefest glance at American academic life shows that this is not so. Wherever the status of schools and universities is organized hierarchically, there will always be competition for places at the top.

Only two solutions offer themselves, and at best they are no more than partial. In the first place, it seems clear that we should make it a much simpler matter than it now is for a man to drop out of the educational system—through boredom or failure—and to re-enter it later, once his mature interest is aroused. Secondly, and more generally, it seems that we should be careful to maintain not one system of entrance to our universities, nor even two, but a diversity of systems, each of them appealing to very different types of person. We should maintain, in other words, a variety of types of examination, not merely a variety of examinations of the same type.

The difficulties which face such a proposal are formidable. First, there are solid political arguments in favour of a simple, unified system of examination and selection for all British universities. This point of view is especially persuasive when one considers the muddle and inefficiencies of the system we now possess ; and, even more persuasive still when we consider that the burden of a multiplicity of examinations is bound to bear most heavily on those grammar schools least able to sustain it. Also, such new examinations are bound to involve a large element of risk. If we admit candidates to university on grounds other than academic (or athletic) ones we are bound, in the early stages especially, to make mistakes —to admit some who are unsuited to University life.

These difficulties have already been experienced at Cambridge. In the academic year 1963-64, the King's Group of Colleges set an Alternative Paper which was, in effect, a psychological projection test in thin disguise—an instrument aimed to elicit imaginativeness unrelated to special academic knowledge. In the first year, some two dozen candidates were admitted on this basis. Certainly, some of these young men are lively and, quite literally, colourful ; whether or not they will contribute to the intellectual lives of their colleges it is at the moment a little too early to say. In the second year, the competition for University places had become so fierce that it was possible to admit not two dozen candidates, but only five or six. There were so many more highly accomplished young men applying for Scholarships and Exhibitions than there were Scholarships and Exhibitions to give, that the risk involved in the Alternative Paper seemed too extreme to take. This present academic year, the Alternative Paper has been dropped.

Despite these difficulties, it seems vital that we should not lose our nerve in the face of democratic arguments about fairness and equality of opportunity, and that we should bear in mind how slight is the justification of conventional academic examinations when they are related to criteria of intellectual accomplishment outside the academic system. Our defence in the face of the errors and inconvenience caused by experimental examinations must be to point out the frailties of the system we are hoping to supersede—that its validity in any but the narrowest academic terms is low, and that its effect on secondary education is regrettable. Whatever is done, it is clear that we must avoid any argument, however plausible, which forces young men and women to spend the formative years of their lives in the mill of increasingly severe competitive examination. Such a system may well be fair, but it is fair at the expense of the intellectual lives of the children it is supposed to serve.

REFERENCES

1. Bloom, B. S. Personal Communication.
2. Holland, J. L. and Kent, L. 1960. The concentration of scholarship funds and its implications for education. *College and University* **35**, 471.
3. Hudson, L. 1960. Degree class and attainment in scientific research. *Brit. J. Psychol.* **51**, 67.
4. Hudson, L. 1961. Arts/science specialization. Unpublished Ph.D. Dissertation, Cambridge University.
5. Hudson, L. 1964. Future open scholars. *Nature* **202**, 834.
6. Hudson, L. 1966. *Contrary Imaginations.* London. Methuen.
7. MacKinnon, D. W. 1962. The nature and nurture of creative talent. *Amer. Psychol.* **17**, 484.
8. Roe, A. 1953. A psychological study of eminent psychologists and anthropologists, and a comparison with biological and physical scientists. *Psychol. Monogr.* **67**, 352.
9. Vernon, P. E. (Ed.). 1957. *Secondary School Selection.* London. Methuen.

SELECTION FOR HIGHER EDUCATION

CONCLUSION

LORD ROBBINS
London School of Economics

WE have been discussing an interesting question and one which is of immense practical importance because the situation with which we are confronted at the present time is, I believe, even more serious than has been suggested in any of the papers read in this section of the Symposium. It is beginning to emerge that the number of applicants of apparent eligibility for university admission likely to be forthcoming in the next few years will be considerably greater than the minimum estimates which were put forward in the Report of the Committee on Higher Education and have been taken by Ministers as a basis for policy. It therefore follows that, if the present degree of efficiency of testing is to continue, a greater and greater number of injustices and inappropriate selections will take place. This, surely, is a very serious thing. It is serious from the point of view of national efficiency, and it is serious also from the point of view of social injustice. Yet where are we? No one in this session has been able to suggest any very satisfactory solution. Dr Hudson provided us with all sorts of extremely cogent reasons for thinking ill of the present system, and I think I agree with nearly everything he says. I think I agree with what Professor Drever said in his remarks upon the unreliability of examiners, and I certainly agree with what Mrs Floud had to say about the pernicious effect the present system of university entrance has on school education. But where do we go from here?

The ordinary intelligence test is palpably unsatisfactory; so are the ordinary examination tests. I personally have a sneaking regard for something of which I was not sure whether Mrs Floud approved or disapproved on balance—first she seemed to me to approve of it, then there came a reference to the *New Yorker* which suggested a slightly disparaging view—I have a sneaking regard for the college entrance examination system in the United States, although one can see that it has considerable limitations. I have a great regard for intelligen interpretation of reports of academic achievement in the schools, and I suspect that, if we had life enough, and time enough, that would be as good a way of choosing people as any other ; but we have not. The numbers are going to become greater. It really is not possible so to organize the lives of university institutions that the detailed and careful process of selection, which is possible in some of the smaller educational institutions, is possible all round.

Therefore, I personally—undeterred by a somewhat sceptical remark made by Dr Hudson—come back to the fact that, until our methods of testing are much more reliable than they seem likely to be in the next twenty or thirty years, we need rather greater elbow-room in university admission. I come back to the view that we need more university places than have been promised hitherto. It is for that reason that I greatly deplore the decision by the present government—of all governments surely the last one would expect to take this line—to draw a sharp line between university education and other forms of higher education and to be determined, apparently, to keep the former down to the practicable minimum.

ASPECTS OF SUBNORMALITY

Chairman: Dr. Brian Kirman

PREGNANCY AND PERINATAL ASSOCIATION WITH MENTAL SUBNORMALITY

JAMES WALKER
Department of Midwifery, University of St Andrews

REPORTING to President Kennedy in 1962, the panel on Mental Retardation stated that [45] in the United States some 3 per cent of the total population was mentally retarded, some severely, the majority only mildly. Some 8 per cent of the mentally retarded required constant care and supervision.

Other speakers in this Symposium will discuss the nature of the syndromes of mental subnormality and the numbers involved; they will no doubt also emphasize the difficulties and problems in estimating the incidence.

THE PROBLEM FOR THE OBSTETRICIAN

We, in obstetrics, are, however, acutely concerned with the criteria to be established when searching for physical or mental deficiencies (to use both terms widely). Studies in our field, designed to elucidate direct causes, or to indicate causal syndrome complexes, can be fully elaborated only if we know what are to be the criteria for normality on the one hand, and for aberration on the other.

The physically or mentally retarded child can be so described only in relation to some level of achievement he is expected to reach at the time of test. If we take an arbitrary level of IQ, or of height, or of physical prowess, we have the comfort of a fixed level which, assuming the accuracy of our techniques, can be measured. This is difficult enough as we know, but why should we necessarily expect, for example, that in the child of intelligent educated professional parents mental retardation should begin only at an IQ of 70? Any IQ below, say, 120 may *in that particular child* be a personal tragedy and be clear evidence, in that child, of pregnancy or perinatal damage lowering his mental ability below his genetic entitlement.

I would suggest that, just as we accept a genetically determined range of ability of all types, so we should accept a wide range of degrees of subnormality, secondary to damage as applicable to the individual child in relation to his own environment and estimated scoring.

There is also the problem in my mind to-day as to how, when searching for pregnancy sequelae, we should correlate children who are physically defective with those who are mentally retarded, or with those who have behavioural or psychotic problems, and with those who have minor damage say to teeth, hearing, eye muscles, or difficulties in interpretation of the printed word. There is a whole range of anomaly, much of which is only now being explored.

As obstetricians, we must be concerned with all aspects of human reproduction. We wish, as you do, to know the truly *genetic* components of our problems, in order that we may give the necessary counsel to the parents. We wish to understand *the social and environmental* components, so that we may attempt in our care programmes to combat deficiencies which are part of these components. We must identify the truly *obstetric or pregnancy* components so that we may prevent damage or minimize its effects. We must foresee the special risks to the neonate so that we can warn our paediatric colleagues and make their task easier.

RISK PREGNANCY

It is seldom realized, except by those directly concerned, that the human, in reproduction, frequently deviates from those physiological standards accepted as normal. In a recent study of ‘ babies at risk ’ in our own city we found (Table 1), using relatively limited criteria, that some 65·2 per cent of all babies born had faced at least one measurable hazard during pregnancy, labour or early neonatal life and that very many had faced several. We cannot then regard ‘ a risk ’ situation as unusual. This has been clearly recognized by wise writers for many years; and the paper of Dr Clement Smith entitled "The valley of the shadow of birth"[54] exemplifies this knowledge.

As in all situations we have of course (*a*) an insult and (*b*) the ability of the individual to cope with the insult at the given time. Fortunately the human foetus can often adapt to combat situations potentially dangerous to himself. He may not however be able to meet the insult by virtue of its intrinsic

TABLE I

RISK BABIES

1075 individual babies, single pregnancies born to 1648 Dundee women in the Royal Infirmary Unit. 65·2 per cent of all deliveries faced the risk situations outlined, some of course more than one.

RISK	PATIENTS	
Threat. abort.	159	
Early illness—pills	151	
Radiology	149	
Antepartum haem.	97	
Folic def. anaemia	80	
Forceps	165	Total 1648—1075 Risk = 65·2 per cent
C/S	85	(Familial TB history excluded)
24 hr. labour	147	
Cord tangle	170	
Foet. dist.	132	
Asphyxia at birth	141	
Virus inf. (contact)	38	

nature, its degree, its duration, or its timing. Some babies, by virtue of pre-existing genetic mal-constitution or because of some intrauterine environmental deficiency, are unable, or less able, to cope with insults that others can surmount.

We too, as well as our paediatric colleagues, have seen much change in techniques of care in recent years. Babies who only yesterday would have died *in utero* are now delivered alive; and babies who would have died in the first few hours are surviving the neonatal period. Modern advance has doubtless increased the number of surviving babies who come from serious risk situations: for example, we now 'save' nearly 60 per cent of all live born babies under 1800 g. at birth;

babies of diabetic mothers rarely die; anoxic babies are resuscitated. Correspondingly by improved standards we have prevented minimum damage to many babies. It is no surprise to me that we are having an unpredicted increase in the number of children capable of and demanding university entrance. Improved obstetric care since the Second World War has contributed largely to this.

PREGNANCY AND PERINATAL ASSOCIATIONS

There are many recognized situations which may be causal in mental subnormality. Some groups and some examples are listed below.

A. GENERAL—Low birth weight [11, 15, 19, 26, 33, 36, 40, 45]
—Maternal relative fertility [16, 39]
—Foetal chromosomal anomaly [20]
—? Maternal dietetic deficiency—? folic acid
—Serological incompatability

B. MATERNAL—(*a*) Infection—Viruses (rubella etc.)
—Cytomegalic inclusion
—Toxoplasmosis
(*b*) Anoxia —Heart disease: respiratory
—CO poisoning: anaesthesia
(*c*) Disease —Hyperthyroid: hypothyroid
—Diabetes
(*d*) Drugs —Thiouracil [3] (low P.B.I.): streptomycin [9]: tetracyclin [8]

C. FOETAL ASPHYXIA—Maternal hypertensive syndromes [17]
—Placental separation early or late [40]
—Cord entanglement

D. FOETAL TRAUMA—Prolonged labour [6, 17, 18, 40]
—Precipitate labour
—Difficult delivery—forceps [17]: breech: manipulation

E. POST-NATAL—Asphyxia [22]
—Hypoglycaemia [41] ? causal
—Hyperglycaemia [70] ? causal
—Hypernatraemia [17]—assoc. with enteritis
—Excessive oxygenation

CEREBRAL PALSY AND MENTAL RETARDATION

Depending on whether the investigators are orientated towards the 'spastic' or 'retarded' child in their study, we find greater or less emphasis placed on pregnancy or perinatal causes. The ' spastic ' investigators [17, 33, 40] tend to find a relatively high incidence of obstetric factors ; in Eastman's [17] series he completely discounts economic status, race and age as being of any significance. In the ' retarded ' studies [15, 16, 19, 36, 37] low birth-weight, with its strong social, economic, familial and genetic associations, tends to hold the main interest.

The Presidential Panel [45] noted that severe mental retardation, usually associated with organic defects, was evenly spread in the population but that milder forms, often not requiring special care and without measurable physical or neurological defect, were heavily concentrated in the poorer socio-economic groups. Drillien [16] (1965) considers that babies born over 2000 g. in weight suffer handicap only because of their environmental disadvantages. Other investigators [19] tend to agree.

THE EFFECT OF FOETAL AGE

It should be clear that the stage of development of the child when the insult is received [59] and the duration of the insult, are of immense importance. It is imperative in any study of prematurity (by weight) that the intra-uterine age of the child at birth be taken as a marker of maturity (there is no better) ; it is also of course necessary to assess the degree of intra-uterine growth of the child by comparing the weight it has reached at birth with an expected weight calculated from measured weights in large series.[65, 66] Length is less useful as the range is scarcely wide enough. Some 40 per cent of babies weighing less than 2500 g. at birth are not prematurely born (Table II), and correspondingly many babies born prematurely are not premature by weight (Table III).

It is clear that the further the birth weight below 2000 g., the greater the likelihood of poor development [16, 36, 37] and the higher the percentage of cases showing a clear association with pregnancy anomaly [16, 65] (Table IV). Moreover, birth-weight below 2000 g. means either birth before the end of the 35th week, which is itself usually associated with pregnancy anomaly (Table V), and with all the neonatal hazards of the small premature [43]; or, if the child is born later, it has suffered a retarded intra-uterine growth, with the possible deficiencies of cerebral development associated with poor

TABLE II

INCIDENCE PER CENT OF PREMATURITY (WEIGHT 2500g. OR LESS) BY GESTATIONAL AGE, INTRA-UTERINE GROWTH
Parity groups in 14,417 legitimate single births to Dundee women, 1960–63 inclusive.

PARITY	1	2	3/4	5+
BORN				
After 37 weeks	43·0	45·0	42·0	30·0
Uncertain	10·0	8·5	11·0	20·0
Before 37 weeks				
Weight below 25th percentile	25·5	22·0	20·5	20·0
Weight above 25th percentile	21·5	24·5	26·5	30·0

(Reproduced from *Gestational Age Size and Maturity*. 1965. Clinics in Developmental Medicine No. 19. Spastics Society, London.)

TABLE III

CLINICAL CAUSES OF LABOUR BEFORE THE END OF THE 36TH WEEK OF GESTATION, ALL DUNDEE WOMEN, 1962

The clear danger of premature labour in first and second twin pregnancies is borne out by the large numbers.

	TOTAL NUMBER	PREMATURE DELIVERY	FROM CLINICAL CAUSE	NOT FROM CLINICAL CAUSE
SINGLE PREGNANCY (No parity difference)				
	3613	110 (3%)	78 (71%)	32* (29%)
TWIN PREGNANCY (102 babies)	51	16	13	3 (6%)
First and second pregnancy :	20	12	10	2
Third and later pregnancy :	31	4	3	1

* Of the 32 babies born prematurely from unknown causes 11 weighed *over* 2500 g.

(Reproduced from the author's Table in *Initiation of Labour* 1963. U.S. Department of Health, Education and Welfare.)

nutrition, specific or general. Many mentally retarded children arise from this latter group.[19]

Intra-uterine growth retardation is a comparatively newly-recognized syndrome [28, 53, 65] which will repay much study of its aetiology and its consequences.

TABLE IV

BIRTH WEIGHT UNDER 1810 g. (4 lbs.). OUTCOME AND CLINICAL CAUSE OF PREMATURITY IN SURVIVORS

Data from 14,417 Dundee Women: single legitimate pregnancies, 1960–63.

Birth weight under 1810 g. (4 lbs.) 246 (27 per cent of all prematures.)

TOTAL	S.B.	1st Week deaths	Survivors	
246	100	82	64	26 per cent total 44 per cent liveborn

Clinical Causes of prematurity in Survivors under 4 lbs. (Represents 0·5–0·8 per cent of total single births).

APH/Th. Abort.	Tox/Mild Tox.	Pyelo.	All Others	SRM/ ?
22	11	7	6	18

(Reproduced from *Gestational Age, Size and Maturity*. 1965. Spastics Society, London.)

TABLE V

PREMATURITY WITHOUT RECOGNIZABLE CLINICAL CAUSE BY INTRA-UTERINE AGE AT BIRTH AND GROWTH WITHIN PARITY GROUPS

14,417 Dundee Women Single legitimate pregnancies, 1960–63.

PARITY	1	2	3/4	5+
BORN				
After 37 weeks	46	50	57	47
Before 37 weeks				
Weight Below 25th percentile	13	10	7	28
Weight Above 25th percentile	27	37	16	23
ALL	30 (per cent)	37 (per cent)	33 (per cent)	35 (per cent)

(Reproduced from *Gestational Age, Size and Maturity*. 1965. Spastics Society, London.)

ASPHYXIA

Windle[69] and Dawes and his collaborators[12, 13,] have contributed much to our knowledge of foetal survival and damage after anoxic insult to the mother. Fraser and Wilks,[22] however, found relatively little long-term damage in children who were over 2500 g. and severely asphyxiated at birth ; minor impairment was common but serious damage rare. It would be very wrong, however, to be too reassured by these findings. It has been shown that the perinatal death-rate[18] and the percentage of neurological anomaly at one year old rise dramatically after labour which lasts more than twelve to eighteen hours. Associated complications such as infection[55] or post-maturity[5, 62, 63] contribute to the risk but the duration itself has biochemical overtones and risks of placental anoxia[6] which are themselves dangerous.

SOCIAL ASPECTS

The Aberdeen School[60] has suggested that, as far as prematurity is concerned, the general health and physique of the mother is more important than the nature of the pregnancy.

Sir Dugald Baird[2] has said, " At this stage of the development of obstetrics in this country the genetic and social inheritance of the baby is of greater importance than the medical complications of pregnancy and delivery." He may be correct if one accepts the statement as relative and in the context in which the statement was made. As pointed out in one Aberdeen study[19] of mentally retarded children, " Low IQ, and domestic and occupational disability are associated with low standards of living and poor nutrition, which lead to stunted growth, poor obstetric performance and low birth-weight ". I would agree that such children start with a disadvantage in that they are neither conceived nor born ' equal ': they also have the poorest maternal intra-uterine environment, the poorest pregnancy and labour care, the poorest postnatal opportunity the poorest environment in which to grow and develop and the highest infancy illness. Maternal iron deficiency,[21] folic acid deficiency,[4, 23, 68] specific protein deficiency, poor heart volume,[46] and maternal infection are all measurably more common.

Prematurity has two components, age and growth. Birth before thirty-seven complete weeks is most often the result of recognized pregnancy anomaly ; birth of the premature, and therefore poorly grown, baby after that time is less often clearly associated with clinically abnormal pregnancy.

All the disadvantages mentioned, however, are specific and often measurable. It is true that with the advent of the well grown, well nourished female of the future some of our problems will disappear, but already, even if we begin only during the pregnancy, we can search out and effectively deal with many of the so-called built-in deficiencies of the lower social groups.

Dugald Baird [1] has suggested that, because of the social composition of this nation, perinatal death-rates below 30 were unlikely, and below 20 utopian. In Aberdeen and even in the industrial City of Dundee, where 23·4 per cent of our pregnant women are under sixty-one inches in height, perinatal mortality rates of 23 and 24 respectively have been obtained in 1963 (Aberdeen) and 1964 (Dundee). What can be done in this regard can be done for reproduction generally, but the cost in effort is very high.

WHAT THEN CAN WE DO?

This presentation, rather than an exposition of clearly defined syndromes, is a plea, first for a change in our attitudes, and, second, for a great extension of our present knowledge.

Ideas to be accepted

1. That all men are neither conceived nor born equal.
2. Recognition by all concerned that conception, pregnancy, birth and neonatal life are beset with hazards. These hazards are admittedly natural, 'acts of God' like drought, flood, tempest, starvation, but they are hazards nonetheless.

3. That those hazards are usually more frequent and more severe in the lower socio-economic groups whose babies are moreover less able to cope with the hazards.

4. That many of those hazards are not mysterious, and that we should define them and learn how to prevent them or minimize their effects.

5. Recognition by obstetricians that a study of national perinatal mortality rates in first and second pregnancies shows that in specialist units up and down the country the best results possible are not yet being achieved. Improvement requires, however, the raising of standards of care and a very great intensification of effort. This can be achieved only by much heavier consultant staffing that has been suggested in recent surveys. It is rarely realized how much effort is necessary to obtain optimum results. Though they themselves may not realize it, most units are grossly understaffed.

General Research

MacKeith [38] has recently suggested intensification of research. Such research is imperative, but I would suggest that much of it should centre on large obstetric units—where the problems do not necessarily begin, but can first be identified—and in centres with fairly stable populations to allow long-term follow up.

1. Follow-up studies of specific risk babies, over a very wide field, for a length of time sufficient to elucidate their status. Purists in research call this 'collecting information'; but we do not even have the information.

2. Retrospective studies of retarded children in an attempt to find previously unrecognized hazards.

3. Further investigation of the perinatal factors associated with minor aberrations of ability even among intelligent children, e.g. minor behaviour anomaly; psychosis; reading defects; visual, auditory and teeth defects, etc.

Immediate perinatal research

1. Intensification of the many studies current in obstetric units of human growth and development over the whole range, from ovarian function through infertility,[25] through abortion,[39] placental function,[10, 14, 24] late pregnancy bleeding,[4] intra-uterine growth,[35] and development and ability to withstand labour.[12, 13, 67]

2. Extension of studies such as those of The Childbirth Research Centre [56] to elucidate the normal behaviour status and the wellbeing and reaction to stress of the foetus in late pregnancy and labour [6, 30] and of the child in the early neonatal period.[7, 31, 41, 44]

Pathology

1. Greater intensification of clinical [48, 59] and pathological studies of the brain lesions of the mentally retarded by modern methods of which those of Schade [49, 50] and Swinyard [58] are examples ; such lesions to be correlated with clinical and causal aetiology.

Lessening the risk situations

1. Prematurity is really an obstetric problem in prevention ; we need much more research.

2. Prematurity, in itself producer of much risk, shows not only a social class correlation, but also a clear correlation with maternal parity greater than four, and age over thirty-five, each factor acting independently (Table VI). A clearly defined drive to limit pregnancies to fewer than five and to discourage childbearing after thirty-five years of age, or a great intensification of care after that parity, or after that age, would pay much dividend.

In the utopian world of the geneticists of the 1930s the natural genophilic impulse would rationalize family size and natural selection [42] ; I am afraid that as an obstetrician I distrust the natural genophilic impulse. Very few women indeed can go on bearing perfect children after the fifth (Table VII) ; very few women want to !

I am certain I have omitted much of importance and have paid inadequate credit to many deserving investigators.

TABLE VI

THE INCIDENCE PER CENT OF PREMATURITY (WEIGHT 2500 g. OR LESS) BY AGE GROUPS WITHIN PARITY GROUPS IN 14,417 LEGITIMATE SINGLE PREGNANCIES
Dundee Women, 1960–63, inclusive.

PARITY/AGE	–19	–24	–29	–34	35+	ALL
1	8·1	6·6	6·7	6·2	13·1	7·0
2	5·5	5·2	3·6	5·3	6·9	4·7
3	8·3	6·2	5·4	4·6	6·9	5·8
4		7·6	6·1	4·6	10·6	6·7
5/6		13·8	8·4	5·6	8·1	7·9
7+			10·1	13·2	7·6	10·2
	7·6	6·3	5·7	5·7	8·3	6·3

(Reproduced from *Gestational Age, Size and Maturity*. 1965 Spastics Society, London.)

TABLE VII

STERILIZATION IN THE POST DELIVERY PERIOD
Dundee Married Women, 1964.

Per cent Post Partum Sterilization/No. of Pregnancy

2nd	3rd	4th	5/6th	7th	ALL
0·7	2	12	27	24	5·2

HIGHEST GROUPS

5/6 Preg.	7+ Preg.
25–29	30–34
41 per cent	42 per cent

My references must be taken only as samples from a vast field. I hope, however, that I have given you some idea of the keen interest of obstetricians in this Symposium and of the important contributions we should be able to make to studies of human reproduction and of mental aberration of any kind.

REFERENCES

1. BAIRD, D. 1960. The evolution of modern obstetrics. *Lancet* ii, 557.
2. BAIRD, D. 1965. In discussion. *Proc. 4th Int. Study Group Child Neurology and Cerebral Palsy*. Spastic Soc.
3. BARNES, C. G. 1962. *Medical Disorders in Obstetric Practice*. Oxford. Blackwell.
4. BLACKLEDGE, D. 1966. *Folic Acid in Pregnancy and Newborn Deficiency States*. (In preparation.)
5. BROWNE, J. McC. 1963. Postmaturity. *Am. J. Obstet. Gyn.* **85**, 573.
6. CALDEYRO-BARCIA, R. *et al.* 1963. The effect of abnormal uterine contractions in a human foetus. *Mod. Probl. Pediat.* **8**, 267.
7. CATHRO, D. M., BIRCHALL, K., MITCHELL, F. L. and FORSYTH, C. C. 1963. The excretion of neutral steroids in the urine of newborn infants. *J. Endocrin.* **27**, 53.
8. CARTER, M. P. and WILSON, F. 1965. Antibiotics in early pregnancy and congenital malformation. *Dev. Med. Child Neurol.* **7**, 353.
9. CONWAY, N. and BIRT, B. D. 1965. Streptomycin in pregnancy—its effect on foetal ear. *Brit. med. J.* ii, 260.
10. COYLE, M. G., GREIG M. and WALKER, J. 1962. Blood progesterone and urinary pregnanediol and oestrogens in foetal death from severe pre-eclampsia. *Lancet* ii, 275.
11. DANN, M., LEVINE, S. Z. and NEW, E. V. 1964. A long-term follow up study of small premature infants. *Pediat.* **33**, 1945.
12. DAWES, G. S., MOTT, J. C., and SHELLEY, H. 1959. The importance of cardiac glycogen for the maintenance of life in foetal lambs and newborn animals during anoxia. *J. Physiol.* **146**, 516.
13. DAWES, G. S., JACOBSON, H. N., MOTT, J. C. and SHELLEY, H. 1960. Some observations on foetal and newborn Rhesus monkeys. *J. Physiol.* **152**, 271.
14. DICZFALUSY, E. 1964. Endocrine functions of the human feto-placental unit. *Fed. Proc.* **23**, 791.
15. DRILLIEN, C. M. 1964. *The Growth and Development of the Prematurely Born Infant*. Edinburgh. Livingstone.
16. DRILLIEN, C. M. 1965. Possible causes of handicap in babies of low birth-weight. *J. Obstet. Gyn. Brit. Comm.* **72**, 993.
17. EASTMAN, N. J., KOHL, S. G., MAISEL, J. E. and KAVALER, F. 1962. The obstetrical background of 753 cases of cerebral palsy. *Obstet. Gyn. Surv.* **17**, 459.
18. EDITORIAL. 1963. Protracted labour. *Lancet* ii, 391.
19. FAIRWEATHER, D. V. I. and ILLSLEY, R. 1960. Obstetric and social origins of mentally handicapped children. *Brit. J. prev. soc. Med.* **14**, 149.
20. FERGUSON-SMITH, M. A. 1960. The techniques of human cytogenetics. *Amer. J. Obstet. Gyn.* **90**, 1035.
21. FIELDING, J., O'SHAUGHNESSY, M. C. and BRUNSTROM, G. M. 1965. Iron deficiency without anaemia. *Lancet* ii, 9.

22. Fraser, M. S. and Wilks, J. 1959. The residual effects of neonatal asphyxia. *J. Obstet. Gyn. Brit. Comm.* **66**, 748.
23. Goodall, H. B. 1961. Megaloblastic anaemia of pregnancy and the puerperium. *Path. Microbiol.* **24**, 682.
24. Greig, M., Coyle, M. G., Cooper, W. and Walker, J. 1962. Plasma progesterone in mother and foetus in the second half of human pregnancy. *J. Obstet. Gyn. Brit. Comm.* **69**, 772.
25. Greig, M. and Macnaughton, M. C. *Maternal and Foetal Utilization of Progesterone.* (In preparation.)
26. Gruenberg, E. M. 1964. *Epidemiological Aspects in Brain Damage in Children.* (Ed. H. G. Birch.) New York. Williams and Wilkins.
27. Gruenwald, P. 1964. The foetus in prolonged pregnancy. *Amer. J. Obstet. Gyn.* **89**, 503.
28. Gruenwald, P. 1964. Infants of low birth weight among 5000 deliveries. *Pediatrics* **34**, 157.
29. Harris, R. and Tizard, J. P. M. 1960. The electroencephalogram in neonatal convulsions. *J. Pediat.* **57**, 501.
30. Hon, E. H. and Lee, S. T. 1963. Electronic evaluation of the foetal heart rate. *Amer. J. Obstet. Gyn.* **87**, 814.
31. Howard, W. F., McDevitt, P. I. and Stander, R. W. 1964. Late cholamine content of initial voided urine of newborn. *Amer. J. Obstet. Gyn.* **89**, 615.
32. Illsley, R., Billewicz, W. Z. and Thomson, A. M. 1954. Prematurity and paid work during pregnancy. *Brit. J. prev. soc. Med.* **8**, 153.
33. Lillienfeld, A. M. and Pasamanick, B. 1955. The association of maternal and fetal factors with the development of cerebral palsy and epilepsy. *Amer. J. Obstet. Gyn.* **70**, 93.
34. Lutwak-Mann, C. and Hay, M. F. 1962. Effects on the early embryo of agents administered to the mother. *Brit. med. J.* ii, 944.
35. McCance, R. A. 1962. Food growth and time. *Lancet* ii, 671.
36. McDonald, A. D. 1962. Neurological and ophthalmic disorders in children of very low birth weight. *Brit. med. J.* i, 895.
37. McDonald, A. D. 1965. Retarded foetal growth. In *Gestational Age, Size and Maturity.* Clinics in Developmental Medicine No. 19. Spastics Society, London.
38. MacKeith, R. I. 1965. Research and the mentally retarded. *Dev. Med. Child Neurol.* **7**, 233.
39. Macnaughton, M. C. 1961. Pregnancy following abortion. *J. Obstet. Gyn. Brit. Comm.* **68**, 789.
40. Mitchell, R. G. 1961. Some Aetiological Considerations. In *Cerebral Palsy*, p. 363. (Ed. J. L. Henderson.) Edinburgh. Livingstone.
41. Neligan, G. A., Robson, E. and Watson, J. 1963. Hypoglycaemia in the newborn: A sequel of intrauterine malnutrition. *Lancet* i, 1282.
42. Osborn, F. 1940. *Preface to Eugenics.* New York. Harper.

43. POLANI, P. E. 1958. Prematurity and cerebral palsy. *Brit. med. J.* ii, 1497.

44. PRECHTL, H. F. R. and BEINTEMA, D. 1964. *The Neurological Examination of the Full-time Newborn Infant.* London. Spastics Society. Heineman.

45. PRESIDENT'S PANEL. 1962. *A Proposed Program for National Action to Combat Mental Retardation.* U.S. Govt. Washington.

46. RAIHA, C. E. 1964. Prematurity perinatal mortality and maternal heart volume. *Guy's Hosp. Rep.* **113**, 96.

47. REID, S. M. 1961. Unexplained prematurity. *J. Obstet. Gyn. Brit. Comm.* **68**, 795.

48. ROSEN, M. G. and SATRAN, R. 1964. Neonatal electroencephalography. *Amer. J. Obstet. Gyn.* **89**, 619.

49. SCHADE, J. P. 1963. Methodology of quantitative brain research. In *Cybernetics and Neural Processes.* (Ed. V. Braitenberg and E. Caianiello.) New York. Academic Press.

50. SCHADE, J. P., VAN BACKLER, H. and COLON, E. 1965. Neuronal parameters in the maturing cerebral cortex. In *Progress in Brain Research.* Amsterdam. Elsevier.

51. SHELLEY, H. J. 1964. Carbohydrate reserves in the newborn infant. *Brit. med. J.* i, 273.

52. SIMON, G. B. 1964. Physical retardation and mental state. *Lancet* ii, 1126.

53. SJÖSTEDT, S., ENGLESON, G. and ROOTH, G. 1958. Dysmaturity. *Arch. Dis. Child.* **33**, 123.

54. SMITH, C. A. 1951. The valley of the shadow of birth. *Amer. J. Dis. Child.* **82**, 171.

55. SMITH, J. A. McC., JENNISON, R. F. and LANGLEY, F. A. 1956. Perinatal infection and perinatal death. *Lancet* ii, 903.

56. SMYTH, C. N. 1965. Exploratory methods for testing the integrity of the foetus and neonate. *J. Obstet. Gyn. Brit. Comm.* **22**, 920.

57. STOTT, D. H. 1965. Congenital indications in delinquency. *Proc. roy. Soc. Med.* **58**, 703.

58. SWINYARD, C. A. and BIRCH, H. G. 1965. Some aspects of postnatal growth, development and function of the human brain pertinent to the natural history of cerebral palsy. In *Gestational Age, Size and Maturity.* Spastics Society, London.

59. TAFT, L. T. and BIRCH, H. G. 1965. Correlative studies of brain injuries and later behavioural aberrations associated with them. In *Gestational Age, Size and Maturity.* Spastics Society, London.

60. THOMSON, A. M. 1961. Prematurity, socio-economic and nutritional factors. *Mod. Prob. Pediat.* **8**, 197.

61. TURNBULL, E. P. N. and WALKER, J. 1956. Outcome of pregnancy following threatened abortion. *J. Obstet. Gyn. Brit. Comm.* **63**, 353.

62. WALKER, J. 1954. Foetal anoxia. *J. Obstet. Gyn. Brit. Comm.* **61**, 162.

63. WALKER, J. 1958. Prolonged pregnancy syndrome. *Amer. J. Obstet. Gyn.* **76**, 1231.
64. WALKER, J. 1960. Obstetric viewpoint on cerebral palsy. *Cereb. Palsy Bull.* **2**, 61.
65. WALKER, J. 1965. Clinical obstetric features of prematurity and intra-uterine growth retardation. In *Gestational Age, Size and Maturity.* Spastics Society, London.
66. WALKER, J. and BILLEWICZ, W. S. 1954. Weight of the human fetus and of its placenta. In *Cold Spr. Harb. Symp. Quant. Biol.* XIX: *The Mammalian Fetus*, p. 39.
67. WALKER, J. and MACNAUGHTON, M. C. (Ed.). 1962. Physical methods of measurement in obstetrics and gynaecology. *J. Obstet. Gyn. Brit. Comm.* **69**, 1029.
68. WELLS, C. E. C. 1965. Clinical neurology and macrocytic anaemia. *Proc. roy. Soc. Med.* **58**, 721.
69. WINDLE, W. F. 1963. Neuropathology of certain forms of mental retardation. *Science* **140**, 1186.
70. WYATT, J. A. and POLLARD, A. C. 1965. Recurrent transient hyperglycaemia in identical twins. *Proc. roy. Soc. Med.* **58**, 690.

ASSESSING THE SIZE OF THE PROBLEM OF SUBNORMALITY

ALBERT KUSHLICK
Wessex Regional Hospital Board, Winchester

THERE are three key problems in assessing the prevalence of subnormality : defining the condition, identifying the affected people, and measuring accurately the population from which they arise, i.e. the population, ' at risk '.

PROBLEMS OF DEFINITION

There is no single morbid condition which causes subnormality and, indeed, a large proportion of people classified as subnormal have no demonstrable pathology ; the definitions vary between different users at the same time and between users of the same type at different times.

Psychometric criterion

The most commonly used measure of general ability is the intelligence score. In terms of this definition, people scoring less than two standard deviations below the population mean are said to be ' subnormal '. Thus, on a test with a mean of 100 and a standard deviation of 15, those people scoring under 70 points are ' subnormal '. Similarly, those scoring lower than three standard deviations below the mean are said to be ' severely subnormal '. On such a test the upper IQ limit of the severely subnormal would be 54 points. This category would include all of the people categorized ' idiot ' and ' imbecile ' in the terminology of the old Mental Deficiency Act. There is, however, no upper IQ limit in the Mental Health Act definition of severe subnormality ; and the average Wechsler IQ of people so classified, who were admitted to hospitals for the subnormal since the Act, was recently found to be 60·4.[43] Those scoring between 55 and 70 points are in terms of the psychometric definition graded 'mildly subnormal'. This category would include those previously classified as feebleminded. The mean Wechsler IQ of people admitted to hospitals for the subnormal was recently found to be 71·4.[43]

Social and educational criteria

The other criteria used to define subnormality are measures of social inadequacy. Some of these, like the Vineland Social Maturity Scale, have been standardized in some places. In the main, however, these criteria are used fairly arbitrarily by clinicians, social administrators, politicians and social planners.

Educational criteria

Among children, a definition of subnormality is needed in order to administer and plan educational facilities. Definitions are needed of categories of handicapped children who may be legally excluded from schools as 'unsuitable' because their behaviour prevents the teacher from achieving his expected role of educating 'normal' children to a prescribed standard. Similarly, definitions are needed of handicapped children who need additional or special forms of education which may be more highly specialized or more expensive in staff and money than the type of education provided for 'normal' children. The history of special education in this country, and the history of mental deficiency legislation, illustrate well how these services have changed over time and how the definitions have followed suit. As provision of education for the handicapped has become more general, children receiving this education have been categorized as educationally subnormal (ESN) rather than mentally defective.

Civil rights criteria

Among adults, criteria are needed to define categories of people, who may be deprived of their rights to determine where and how they are going to live and whether they are going to conceive and care for their own children.

Criteria are also needed to define those adults who should be relieved by society of the social responsibility to maintain themselves financially and socially. The history of mental deficiency legislation in this country illustrates the extent to which these definitions have changed over time. The Mental Health Act (1959), for example, attempts to give more precise descriptions than the Mental Deficiency Act (1913) and to limit more exactly the section of the population liable, on account of their subnormality, to be legally detained in institutions.[19]

Clinical criteria

Finally, there are clinical definitions ; and these are of two types. First, there are the overt, morbid, clinical entities, which are so often accompanied by social and educational handicaps in affected people that the morbid condition is virtually equivalent to subnormality.

Of these, mongolism (Down's Syndrome) is the most important numerically, but the rarer conditions like gargoylism and cranial abnormalities can be included in this category.

The second major group of clinical categories of subnormality includes children and adults, with or without pathological abnormalities, who manifest delay in achieving the expected stages of motor, social and intellectual functioning. Some of these criteria are standardized and overlap with the biological or psychometric criteria ; others are more arbitrary and empirical and overlap with the social and educational criteria outlined above. The overlap between the clinical and the social or educational criteria arises from the fact that society has, to a large extent, entrusted the medical profession with the right to categorize children who will be either excluded from, or given, special services and the adults who will be either deprived of civil rights, or relieved of adult social responsibilities.

As each classification may have some merit, the investigator must first examine the characteristics of the people already classified as subnormal by the agencies dealing with the problem, i.e. the 'administrative prevalence' of subnormality. Then the people classified can be described in terms of all the available criteria, psychometric, clinical, social and educational. The number of people known to the administrative agencies depends to a large extent on the quality and quantity of the services provided. In order to find the 'true' prevalence the investigator must identify those people who are not known to the agencies as subnormal. He is therefore obliged to take one or more of the possible criteria and seek out those people who fall within the chosen limits. Most investigators have attempted, in large population surveys, to measure the 'true prevalence' among children of school age, since they provide what is virtually a 'captive population'.

Space does not permit me to discuss the third problem, that of identifying the population 'at risk' which comprises the denominator in the calculation of the prevalence rates.

Classification used in this paper

In this paper the term 'subnormal' will be used to include all grades of subnormality. The terms 'idiot', 'imbecile' and 'severely subnormal' will be used to mean people scoring IQs of under 50. The terms 'feebleminded' and 'mildly subnormal' will be used interchangeably to mean people of IQ over 50 who are classified as subnormal.

There are empirical justifications for using these criteria and these will now be described.

IDENTIFICATION

The prevalence and prognosis of severe subnormality

In England about 3·7 per thousand of the people who survive to the age of fifteen to nineteen are likely to be severely subnormal. Kushlick [21] examined the records of all mental defectives known on 1st January 1961 to the Mental Health Department in Salford, a northern English industrial city of 153,000 people. Goodman and Tizard [14] examined the records of all mental defectives known in 1961 to the Mental Health Department of the County of Middlesex with a population of 2,231,100. They also collected details of children of IQ under 50 who were of school age but were not known

TABLE I

PREVALANCE OF SUBNORMALITY BY AGE AND GRADE

	Grade				All Grades				
	Severely S/N		Mildly S/N						
	Salford 1961 [21]	England † 1926-29 [26]	Salford 1961 [21]	England † 1926-29 [26]	Salford 1961 [21]	England 1926-29 (From Penrose [26, 34])	Baltimore 1936 [25]	Onondaga 1955 [30]	Rural Sweden 1951 [1]
0–4	0·89	0·69	0·15	0·51	1·13	1·2	0·7	4·5	12·5
5–9	1·62	3·09	0·36	11·41	1·98	15·5	11·8	39·4	18·4
10–14	2·55	4·35	0·29	21·25	2·84	25·6	43·6	77·6	37·2
15–19	3·62	2·84	8·63	7·96	12·27	10·8	30·2	—	14·2
20–29	3·44	2·07	4·16	6·33	7·66	8·4	7·2 ‡	—	19·7
30–39	3·77	1·49	1·83	4·21	5·59	5·7	8·1 ‡	—	22·7
40–49	2·47	1·22	2·56	4·18	5·04	5·4	8·3 ‡	—	17·7
50–59	1·70	0·90	1·04	4·00	2·83	4·9	6·4 ‡	—	17·6
60	0·52	0·48	0·60	2·42	1·13	2·9	2·6 ‡	—	8·4
							1·9 ‡		
TOTALS	2·24	1·87	2·057	6·73	4·38	8·6	12·2	—	17·4

† Calculated from Lewis [26] Tables 17 (A) and (C) ; and from Penrose [34] p. 23.
‡ Age groups are 20–24 ; 25–34 ; 35–44 ; 45–54 ; 55–64 ; 65.

to the Mental Health Department, because they were still attending schools within the ordinary educational system, private schools and private homes. Kushlick [22] examined the records of all mental defectives known on 1st July 1963 in the area served by the Wessex Regional Hospital Board. The three county boroughs, Southampton, Portsmouth and Bournemouth, and the three counties, Hampshire, Dorset and the Isle of Wight, had a total population of 1,740,000 people. The

TABLE II

PREVALENCE OF IQ UNDER 50 IN AGE-GROUPS WHERE ALL SUBJECTS ARE LIKELY TO BE KNOWN

	AGE-GROUP	TOTAL IQ UNDER 50 per thousand	MONGOL per thousand
England and Wales (Lewis [26])			
1926–29 Urban	7–14	3·71	0·34
Rural		5·61	N/K
Middlesex (Goodman and Tizard [14])			
1960	7–14	3·45	1·14
1960	10–14	3·61	N/K
Salford (Kushlick [21])			
1961	15–19	3·62	0·90
Wessex (Kushlick [22])			
1964 County Boroughs	15–19	3·54	1·15
Counties	15–19	3·84	1·18
Onondaga [30]			
1955	5–17	3·6	N/K
Baltimore (Lemkau *et al.*[25])			
1936	10–14	3·3	N/K
Rural Sweden (Åkesson [1])			
1959	All ages	5·8	0·03

records were obtained from the mental health departments of the Local Health Authorities, the psychiatric hospitals for the subnormal and the mentally ill, and from registered private homes serving the Region. The prevalence of severe subnormality found in these surveys in comparable age groups is shown in Table II. The rates for both urban and rural areas are very similar.

Prevalence rates of severe subnormality in the USA are similar to those found in this country, but differences in survey methods render comparisons with English results difficult.

The English studies suggest that distinct clinical entities are now contributing similar proportions to this condition. Thus, Table II also shows that the prevalence of mongolism at the age of fifteen to nineteen is very similar in all the surveys ; most mongols are severely subnormal, although our findings in Wessex suggest that just over 10 per cent of mongols have IQs of over 50. Mongolism at present accounts for about one quarter of all cases of severe subnormality in this age group.

The means of identifying severely subnormal subjects is similar in all industrialized countries. In the United Kingdom most of them are excluded from school because they are deemed by teachers, head teachers, educational psychologists and school medical officers to be 'unsuitable for education' in the ordinary school system. They are then notified to the Mental Health Department of the Local Health Authority which becomes responsible for their care and training.

In the United Kingdom nearly all severely subnormal people who have survived to the age group of fifteen to nineteen have been notified to Mental Health Departments. Kushlick [21] found that only a very small proportion of these subjects were notified for the first time after the age of nineteen. The reason for this appears to lie in the prognosis of people with severe subnormality. Only about 10 per cent of these subjects are able to hold employment in open industry.[44] The remaining 90 per cent appear at the present time to remain permanently dependent economically, and for this reason become known to the social agencies dealing with subnormality. This has been shown directly by follow-up studies and indirectly from other evidence. For example, Table I shows that the age-distribution of severe subnormality remains fairly constant between adolescence and middle-age, suggesting that these people are in need of special services for the whole of their lives. In contrast, the rates for mild subnormality decline sharply after adolescence, suggesting that their incapacity is of a temporary nature related to educational difficulties during the period of school age.

It has also been shown that nearly all severely subnormal subjects who survive childhood are eventually admitted to hospitals for the subnormal. It is known that the waiting list for admission to these hospitals consists largely of the severely subnormal, and that once they are admitted they are seldom, if ever, discharged.

The prevalence and prognosis of mild subnormality

The IQ range 50–70 or 75 has been suggested as diagnostic of the grade of mild subnormality. This has not proved useful, either clinically or administratively. There are many people in this IQ range who are never dealt with as subnormal and who do not appear to have problems arising from their low intelligence, and there are people of IQ well over 70 who are being dealt with by the services for the subnormal. In the United Kingdom there has never been an upper psychometric limit to this degree of subnormality. On a test standardized to give a mean of 100 and standard deviation of 15 the proportion of the population scoring between 50 and 70 would be nearly 20/1000. In the Salford survey the highest prevalence rate for mild subnormality was found among those aged fifteen to nineteen ; it was 8·6/1000, or under half the rate expected on the criterion of IQ alone (see Table I). Nor is the IQ level the sole determinant of who is to be classified as Educationally Subnormal (ESN) and given special education within the ordinary school system. The total number of children in special schools seldom exceeds half of the 2 per cent to be expected, if all children of IQ 50–70 were to attend. Moreover, the Chief Medical Officer's Report for 1962 [17] shows that about 40 per cent of children in the special schools scored over 70.

Unlike the severely subnormal, most of whom are excluded from the ordinary school system, the majority of the mildly subnormal first become so classified in this country when they are notified by the Education Authority to the Mental Health Department as in need of supervision on leaving school. Thus, 90 per cent of the mildly subnormal people referred to Salford Mental Health Department between 1948 and 1960 were notified between the ages of fifteen and nineteen.[21] This also explains why Mental Health Department Registers have very few mildly subnormal people aged under fifteen and why there is a sharp rise in their numbers in the age group fifteen–nineteen (Table I).

There is much evidence from both follow-up studies and the age distribution of the condition (Table I) that, unlike severe subnormality, mild subnormality is a temporary incapacity related largely to educational difficulties experienced at school. After leaving school, the majority of these people become socially and economically independent and are indistinguishable from the rest of the community. Only a minority of the mildly subnormal subjects are ever admitted to hospital: they are distinguishable from their peers mainly by their experiences of being reared in profoundly broken homes and by multiple placements in residential institutions or foster homes.[41] These findings suggest that their social inadequacies may arise from a lack of social skills, normally acquired by children within their own families,[33] and from the possession of social skills learned in and appropriate to large authoritarian institutions, but which prove dysfunctional when the subjects have to adjust to the complexities of social relationships outside institutions.[7, 13]

Inconstancy of the IQ

It has also been shown that people categorized as mildly subnormal or educationally subnormal continue to make IQ increments for some years after it is believed that IQ growth is complete.[5, 6, 41] This observation questions the validity of the IQ as an assessment of innate 'intelligence' among the mildly subnormal, and it complicates further any attempt to measure the prevalence of mild subnormality by the criterion of IQ.

In the first place, this phenomenon appears to be characteristic of mild subnormality in the absence of brain damage, and may partly explain the good prognosis of these subjects after they leave school. It suggests that the ability of the mildly subnormal to profit from education may indeed improve from the time they leave school, and emphasizes their need for adult education on leaving school.

While the data show that most of the severely subnormal subjects who do not die at an early age are eventually admitted to hospitals, this should not be taken to mean that this is the only or the best way to cater for their or their families' needs.

It demonstrates merely that they appear, at present, to have a type of incapacity requiring a form of special provision for the whole of their lives, in contrast to the mildly subnormal, whose incapacities and needs are largely temporary. Second, the respective prognoses illustrated for the two grades are valid only for large numbers of cases ; whereas the prognosis in an individual case requires the skilled consideration of many factors other than the IQ. Third, while it is clear that those in the IQ category over 50 merge imperceptibly with the community at large, the medium grade IQ range (20–49) contains within it a wide variation of capacity, which overlaps at the upper end with that of the category of IQ over 50.

The causes of mental defect

The primary cause of intellectual handicap among the severely subnormal appears to be observable pathology in the brain, which is almost always present [8] ; however, in only a small proportion of the cases is a definite cause known. Berg and Kirman [3] examined the records of imbeciles and idiots, who were consecutive admissions to the Fountain Hospital (Table III). A definite causal factor was found in only 9·5 per cent of cases, for example iso-immunization and prematurity kernicterus, tuberculous and influenzal meningitis, post-immunization encephalopathy and recessive genetic conditions such as phenylketonuria, galactosaemia and cerebral lipoidosis. Mongols account for 23 per cent of the subjects. In 31 per cent, however, no causal factor was identifiable. There are no comparable intensive studies of the clinical and neuropathological lesions among complete populations of IQ 50–70. About a quarter of the subjects selected in ESN surveys appear to have clinical signs of brain damage or sensory defects. The remainder appear clinically normal.[41]

Social class and mental subnormality

It has long been known that parents of severely subnormal children are evenly distributed among all the social strata of industrial society, while those of mildly subnormal subjects come predominantly from the lower social classes.

There is now evidence which suggests that mild subnormality in the absence of abnormal neurological signs (epilepsy, electroencephalographic abnormalities, biochemical abnormalities, chromosomal abnormalities or sensory defects) is virtually confined to the lower social classes. Indeed, there is

TABLE III

AETIOLOGICAL FACTORS IN 200 CONSECUTIVE ADMISSIONS [3]

GROUP A: DUE TO KNOWN FACTOR	19 (9·5 per cent)
1. Environmental:	
Kernicterus due to rhesus incompatibility	6
Kernicterus of prematurity	1
Meningitis, tuberculosis	4
Meningitis, influenzal	1
Pertussis immunization	1
2. Genetic:	
Phenylketonuria	3
Cerebral lipoidosis:	
Amaurotic family idiocy	1
Unclassified	1
Galactosaemia	1
GROUP B: PROBABLY DUE TO FACTOR INDICATED	8 (4 per cent)
1. Environmental:	
Maternal rubella	1
Therapeutic irradiation of mother	1
Thiouracil treatment of mother	1
Septicaemia, neonatal	1
Septicaemia with sinus thrombosis	1
Gastro-enteritis with coma	1
Encephalitis	1
2. Genetic:	
Hypoglycaemia	1
GROUP C: OTHER FACTORS IMPLICATED	111 (55·5 per cent)
1. Environmental:	
Birth trauma: probable	27
Birth trauma: possible	9
2. Genetic:	
Family history of mental retardation	18
Family history of mental disorder, epilepsy, or other neurological abnormality	10
3. Unknown:	
Mongolism	46
Sturge-Weber syndrome	1
GROUP D: NO FACTORS SUGGESTED	62 (31 per cent)

evidence that almost no children of higher social class parents have IQ scores of less than 80, unless they have one of the pathological processes mentioned above. This has been observed among ESN children, children referred to the school psychological service and among eleven-plus test results.[42] The results of the Scottish Mental Survey of 1947 also confirm these findings.[39]

There is now much evidence that this reflects on the one hand characteristics of the lower working class subculture already discussed during this Symposium, and on the other the social and material deprivations suffered by the lower social classes, particularly in the use of medical and educational services ; these disadvantages have now been well documented both in official documents and in the professional literature.[2, 4, 9, 10, 16, 31, 35]

IS THE PREVALENCE OF SUBNORMALITY INCREASING OR DECREASING?

Severe subnormality

Differences between current prevalence rates and those found by Lewis [26] in his classical survey of 1929 must be interpreted cautiously, because the expansion of services for the subnormal may have rendered the identification of such cases easier now than in 1926–29, and the standardization of the IQ tests used then and now may differ. Such comparisons suggest that, in spite of increased survival-rates of mongolism, the prevalence of severe subnormality has fallen since 1929. The apparent fall in prevalence may, however, be masking a real increase in severe subnormality as we now see it, i.e. characterized by permanent severe incapacity. Thus, Goodman and Tizard [14] (Table II), showed that the prevalence of severe subnormality in the age group seven to fourteen had decreased from Lewis's figure of 3·71/1000 in the urban areas to 3·45/1000 in Middlesex in 1961 ; in the same period, the prevalence of mongolism increased from 0·34 to 1·14/1000. They cautiously interpreted their findings as reflecting an apparent decrease in the prevalence of non-mongol severe subnormality. Possible explanations for this apparent decrease are improved obstetric standards and reduction of infectious diseases. The prevalence of severe subnormality in the age group fifteen to nineteen in Salford in 1961 was 3·62/1000 and in the Wessex County Boroughs in 1963 it was 3·54/1000. The apparent decrease in the rural areas was even higher. Lewis's 1926–29 rate in the rural areas was 5·61/1000 in the age-group seven–fourteen, compared with the 1963 rate of 3·84/1000 in the Wessex Counties in the age-group fifteen–nineteen.

On the other hand, there is also evidence of an increase in prevalence. Table I shows that the total prevalence rates of severe subnormality and the age-specific rates for those aged fifteen and over were higher in Salford in 1961 than those found in Lewis's Survey. Kushlick[21] showed that in Salford the total prevalence of idiots had increased between 1948 and 1960 by 83 per cent, and that of imbeciles by 38 per cent. Possible reasons for the increase are the observed increased survival rate of mongols and hydrocephalics, and the new problem created by the survival of very low birth-weight prematures and children with tuberculous meningitis, now the major cause of severe subnormality next to mongolism.

The author favours this explanation of the paradox: that Lewis's sample in the age-group seven–fourteen might have included a large proportion of non-brain-damaged subjects with temporary incapacities similar to the subject with mild subnormality, whereas most of the children of IQ under 50 in the recent surveys are brain-damaged and permanently handicapped. Table I shows that the prevalence of severe subnormality in Salford remains fairly constant up to the age of forty, suggesting that these subjects continue to require supervision in or out of hospital until they die. However, the 1926–29 rates, like those for the subjects with mild subnormality, drop immediately after school-leaving age. This suggests that some of Lewis's severely subnormal subjects in the age-group seven to fourteen might, on leaving school, have adjusted sufficiently well to the demands of society, and that Lewis's rates in the subsequent quinquennium 15–19, are a truer reflection of the prevalence of severe subnormality characterized by permanent incapacity. It is, of course, possible, as Lewis himself suggests, that there were large numbers of severely subnormal people aged fifteen to nineteen unknown to the agencies he used as sources. Such agencies as the Labour Exchange and the Public Assistance Committee might have been expected to know of the large numbers of unemployed imbeciles anticipated from the difference in rates between the age-groups seven to fourteen and fifteen to nineteen ; the unemployment rate was very high at the time of his survey. We are, alas, unable to compare the distribution of clinical conditions found among Lewis's subjects with that observed in recent surveys. Lewis's clinical data were not analysed for his report. They were carefully stored in his bank in the hope that they would be safe until he had time to analyse them. The bank was bombed during the war and the data were lost completely.

Mild subnormality

Because of the problem of definition it is much more difficult to estimate the trends of mild subnormality. The results of the Scottish Survey of IQs of eleven-year-old children showed, if anything, a fall in the proportion of low scorers between 1932 and 1947. Provision for ESN children has increased over the years, but this reflects only improvements in a service which has always been lacking.

The proportion of mildly subnormal people in hospitals for the subnormal has decreased since 1938, and there is evidence that the absolute number may also have declined since 1951.[23a] The discharge rate of subnormal patients doubled in 1956 and has remained at this level ever since.[36, 37] The length of stay in hospital of people discharged has also decreased.[38] Unless there is a high re-admission rate, the numbers of chronic mildly subnormal patients in hospital should continue to fall.

The proportion of legally detained patients is now comparatively small. On 31 December 1963, in England and Wales 5,323 (8·2 per cent) of the 65,000 subnormal people in psychiatric hospitals were legally detained and 1,112 (1·7 per cent) were detained in the special security hospitals, Rampton and Moss Side.[32] There has been very little systematic study of this problem. It is likely that, if the recent liberalizing of custodial regimes in the hospitals for the mentally ill is adopted by the hospitals for the subnormal, the difficulty of meeting the requirements of the minority of the subjects who need custodial care may be passed on to the state security institutions. Systematic epidemiological studies into the reasons for, and the effects of, custodial care of subnormal subjects are urgently needed.

At present in Great Britain, people of limited capacity are, like everyone, benefiting from reasonably full employment. If, however, the introduction of automation is allowed to create problems of mass unemployment, as it has done in the United States, clearly the mildly subnormal and other people in the social classes from which they come will be severely hit.

THE USE OF THESE DATA

The following are some important qualifications to observe in assessing the epidemiological data on severe subnormality:

1. The prevalence and prognosis of the condition are to some extent determined by the available services. Therefore we shall not know the true extent or prognosis of these people until, first, the existing shortage has been met and sufficient facilities are available to cover all the needs of the affected people and their families, and second, the methods of management have been evaluated and affected people have been given the benefit of the best of those available. We may thus now be seeing not a 'true' prognosis, but the results of the complications of the underlying organic process.

2. Some of these complications are, and others may be, avoidable. An obvious example is the retarding effect on emotional development, speech and verbal intelligence observed among children in large institutions.[27, 40, 46] Moreover, the failure to provide adequate early counselling and relief to the parents of affected children may, by causing family tension, retard the child's development. Furthermore, we do not know the educational potential of these children in the hands of skilled qualified teachers, or even with the use

of such aids as teaching machines. The present policy, in England and Wales, of excluding many of these children from the ordinary educational system, and the reluctance of many child-guidance clinics to accept responsibility for their long-term care may well be to the disadvantage of the children.

3. The overall prognosis for the severely subnormal is relatively poor, but even with the present facilities, their potential social and intellectual development in adulthood ranges widely, from that of infantile behaviour to the ability to work in sheltered or open industry. This is particularly true of mongolism. Thus, Dunsdon *et al.*[11] found that 6–7 per cent of mongols scored IQs of over 45 and that 1–2 per cent scored 55 and over. Our own findings in Wessex suggest that just over 10 per cent of mongols aged fifteen–nineteen had IQs of over 50. There is also growing evidence that a proportion of phenylketonurics (even untreated) may have normal or near-normal intelligence.[12] Moreover, while very experienced paediatricians can predict in early infancy, with about 60 per cent accuracy, the non-mongol children who will have IQs of under 50, the substantial remainder will do much better, and it is virtually impossible to predict the final development of individual children within the IQ range under 50.[20]

These facts emphasize the necessity for providing at the earliest possible stage the very best facilities for children suspected of being subnormal.

SERVICES FOR THE SUBNORMAL

Can these data be used to plan services? The factors associated with mild subnormality suggest that this condition might be reduced if a specially high standard of services—antenatal care, maternal and child welfare, medical and educational (both pre-school and adult)—were to be provided for people in unskilled and semi-skilled working-classes who constitute the 'vulnerable group' as far as this condition is concerned. Even the provision of normally adequate facilities would probably be effective in achieving a reduction. Our prevalence data, however, offer little more than an empirical guide to the planning of such services.

On the other hand, our information on severe subnormality offers little hope at present of substantially reducing these conditions. However, the consistent data on the 'true' prevalence of severe subnormality among children enable us, first, to assess the extent to which the services are meeting the needs and, second, to evaluate objectively the merits and demerits of different types of services for these people.

The extent to which we are meeting the needs of the severely subnormal

In Table IV we have an arbitrary population of 100,000, with an annual birth rate of 16/1000 (the average in England and Wales in the past sixteen years).

TABLE IV

CALCULATION OF THE NUMBER OF CHILDREN OF IQ UNDER 50 WHO WILL BE BORN IN A PERIOD OF 16 YEARS IN A POPULATION OF 100,000

Population	100,000
Birth rate per year	16/1000
Births per year	1,600
Births in 16 years	25,600
Subjects of IQ under 50	$3{\cdot}7 \times 25{\cdot}6 \doteqdot 100$

Our arbitrary population has a minimum of six new cases of severe subnormality every year (3·7 per 1·6 thousand). Table V shows that over a five-year period, there are about thirty cases. Because our rates are based on survivors to the age of ten to nineteen years, we can assume that all of these children survive to the age of sixteen. There would be a minimum of nearly 100 children aged 0–15 in our population; thirty aged 0–4 and sixty-six aged 5–15. About one in six of these children are probably idiots, scoring IQs lower than 20.[21] The number of cases who have diagnosable clinical conditions is estimated from the proportions found by Berg and Kirman [3] in their hospital survey.

Only a quarter of the cases will have clinical conditions diagnosable at birth or shortly after. However, a substantial proportion of the remaining three-quarters will have signs of a central nervous system disorder such as epilepsy, cerebral palsy, defects of hearing or vision and behaviour disorders. They will also show developmental delay. The demands on a diagnostic service for our population, if all severely subnormal children are to be detected early, will be many more than six new cases a year because it would also be caring for those children with such abnormalities who will subsequently develop normally.

TABLE V

EXPECTED PREVALENCE OF SEVERE SUBNORMALITY AMONG CHILDREN IN A POPULATION OF 100,000 WITH A BIRTH-RATE OF 16/1000

AGE	NO. OF CHILDREN	MINIMUM NO. OF SEV. SUB.	MONGOLS	IDIOTS	PKU	TBM	RH.	RUB.
0–4	8,000	30	8 (+1)	5				
5–15	17,600	66	17 (+2)	11				
Total:	25,600	96	25 (+3)	16	1	3	1	1

Figures in parenthesis are the numbers of mongols of IQ 50 and over.

RH = Rhesus incompatibility
RUB = Rubella encephalopathy

Table VI shows the extent to which the MHDs are aware of the existing cases and the way in which the services are being used. Only four of the thirty severely subnormal children aged 0–4 are known to the Mental Health Department. One is in an institution, one attends a day training centre from his home, and two live at home, where they receive only visits from a mental welfare officer. At least some of the remaining twenty-six are probably known to their general practitioners, to paediatricians and health visitors ; but this needs further investigation.

Forty-seven of the expected sixty-six severely subnormal children aged 5–15 years were known to the Mental Health Department. The remaining nineteen were not yet known to the MHD because they were still at school. Our experience is that most of these school children attend special schools from the age of seven. Sixteen of those known to the Mental

Health Department are in institutions, twenty-two attend day training centres from home, seven live at home and receive no training. In all, three of the children are on the waiting list for admission to hospital.

TABLE VI

OBSERVED PREVALENCE OF SEVERE SUBNORMALITY KNOWN TO MHDs AMONG CHILDREN IN A POPULATION OF 100,000

Wessex Region (excluding Wiltshire)—1.7.63. Rates per 100,000

Age	HC	HC + TC	Inst.	Other	Total	Total expected	SSN not known to MHD
0–4	2	1	1	—	4	30	26
5–15	7	22	16	2	47	66	19
Total	9	23	17	2	51	96	45

HC = Home Care, not receiving training.
HC+TC = Home Care and attending Training Centre.
Inst. = Hospital Care and Hostels.
Other = Guardianship, Approved Schools, Foster Homes.

Table VII, which gives the prevalence of *all* grades of subnormal children known to the Mental Health Departments in our population of 100,000, shows that there were also thirteen mildly subnormal children known—six were receiving training in MHD training centres, three were in institutions and four were apparently at home and not attending training centres. This table also shows that a total of thirteen children were at home not attending training centres. The reason that

TABLE VII

OBSERVED PREVALENCE OF ALL GRADES OF SUBNORMALITY KNOWN TO MHDs AMONG CHILDREN IN A POPULATION OF 100,000

Wessex Region (excluding Wiltshire) 1.7.63. Rates per 100,000.

Age	HC	HC + TC	Inst.	Other	Total
0–4	3	1	2	—	6
5–15	10	28	18	2	58
Total	13	29	20	2	64

those who have been excluded from school are not receiving training is that they are considered too severely retarded or too physically handicapped for the existing training centres. Special-care facilities will be needed for these children. Thus 42 (13+29) junior training centre places will be required to take all children excluded from school. In 1962 in England and Wales, 30 per cent of Local Health Authorities had more than fifty places per 100,000 population, and in 1972, 53 per cent plan to do so.[18]

Experimental evaluation of services for the severely subnormal

Prevalence data of this type might also be used to evaluate the many different types of service we are now providing, or may provide in the future. Developments in services cannot take place everywhere simultaneously. An area where a new type of service is set up, therefore, becomes a potential experimental area and its facilities might fruitfully be evaluated against the results achieved by the traditional type of service in a demographically comparable control area. A research team of people with the required skills would measure in both experimental and control areas, the progress of the affected people, the level of problems among their families, the administrative problems as well as the costs involved. They would also study systematically the quality of the relationships in the different types of service.

In this way, for example, we hope to evaluate in parts of the Wessex Region a new form of residential provision for severely subnormal children. Table VII shows that twenty children from our population of 100,000 are already in institutions for the mentally subnormal ; a further three are on the waiting list. The institutions are often large, and nearly always a long distance from the children's families. We already know the proportion of various types of disabilities among these children (Table VIII).

In our experimental area we hope to provide, in small units, twenty-five residential places for these children in the areas to which they belong and to evaluate in this way the comparative merits of these two types of care. A description of these plans has been published.[23]

Methods developed successfully in this field will be useful in evaluating other forms of medical care. The technical problems of experimental design for any morbid condition would have much in common, and measures of social and family problems caused by a chronically handicapped member could be used over a wide range of medical conditions. There are already impressive examples of crossfertilization of techniques evolved in the field of mental subnormality to other medical problems.[15, 45] In the course of these studies much fundamental information on subnormality will also be collected.

TABLE VIII

SOCIAL AND PHYSICAL INCAPACITIES AND BEHAVIOUR DISORDERS (PERCENTAGES) AMONG ALL WESSEX (EXCLUDING WILTSHIRE) SUBNORMAL CHILDREN AGED 15 AND UNDER IN RESIDENTIAL CARE ON 1ST JULY 1963 BY PLACE OF CARE

Place of Care	Incontinent only	Incontinent & bedfast.	Incontinent & Behaviour diff's.	Behaviour Difficulties only	None of these	Total (Percentages)	N
Registered Private Homes	15	36	9	6	33	99	66
Hospitals	23	24	15	12	25	99	242
Whole Region	22	26	13	11	28	100	321*

* 13 cases were in Local Authority Hostels.

Penrose has described several ways in which the severely subnormal have contributed to our understanding of the society from which they are alienated. In these experimental studies they would be making a further contribution and one from which, we hope, they might benefit directly.

Until we understand what environments are the most favourable for developing the abilities of people with different handicaps, and until we have both provided the affected people with the best possible environments and removed the known unfavourable factors, any estimate of the respective contributions of the biological or organic endowment on the one hand and the environment of the other, to the potential of handicapped people—even the severely subnormal—must remain highly speculative.

TABLE IX

Prevalence of Known Subnormality among Adults aged 16 and over by Grade and Place of Care on 1st July 1963

Wessex Region (excluding Wiltshire).

IQ	Area	HC	HC+TC	Inst.	Other	Total	Waiting List	Population in thousands 1961 Census
Under 50	Counties	33	18	73	3	127	2	1,172
	County Boroughs	32	20	76	5	133	4	574
	Total	32	19	74	4	129	3	1,746
Over 50	Counties	62	10	55	18	145	1	
	County Boroughs	55	9	51	11	126	2	
	Total	60	9	53	16	138	1	
Not known	Counties	1	—	5	1	8	—	
	County Boroughs	4	—	4	—	9	—	
	Total	2	—	5	1	8	—	
Total	Counties	96	29	133	22	280	3	
	County Boroughs	91	29	131	17	268	6	
	Total	94	29	132	20	275	4	

Other = Guardianship, Approved Schools, Residential Employment, etc.

DISCUSSION

Dr Kushlick, when asked to enlarge on the association of prematurity with low intelligence, said:

If one defines as 'premature' children of birth weight under 5½ lbs. (2,500 gm), the available evidence suggests that the association observed between low birth weight and mild subnormality (IQ 50–69) is due to the common factor of low social class, whereas there is good evidence that severe subnormality (IQ under 50) is associated with very low birth weight, independently of social class.

Only among children of birth weight under 3 lbs. is the mean IQ lowered (Douglas, 1960 *; McDonald, 1964 †). The proportion of these children who are mildly subnormal (IQ 50–69) appears to be increased, among the boys, from the expected 29/1000 [39] to the observed 41/1000. Among the girls, the rate observed is only 11/1000 (McDonald †). However, among girls born to fathers of social classes I and II McDonald found no decline in the mean IQ even of children with birth weights of less than 3 lbs. Both Douglas and McDonald demonstrated that within each social class the mean IQ of children of birth weights under 4 lbs. and without gross physical abnormalities was not significantly lower than the mean IQ of mature children.

Drillien (1961 ‡) has found within all social classes that the mean IQ of children of birth weight 3½ lbs. and less was lower than the mean IQ of mature children. However, she included the IQs of grossly abnormal children in her computation of the mean IQ whereas McDonald and Douglas did not. Douglas, McDonald and Drillien all agree that at every level of birth weight under 4 lbs. (and Douglas shows that at any level of birth weight) the mean IQ of children without gross abnormality declines from high to low social class. The

* Douglas, J. W. B. 1960. *Brit. med. J.* 1, 1008.

† McDonald, Alison D. 1964. Intelligence of children of very low birth weight. *Brit. J. of prev. and soc. Med.* **18**, 59-73.

‡ Drillien, C. M. 1961. A longitudinal study of the growth of prematurely and maturely born children. Part VII. *Arch. Dis. in Child* **36**, 233-240.

incidence of babies weighing less than 5½ lbs. or 2500 gm. rises from higher to lower social classes.[2, 35]

On the other hand McDonald showed that of single children of birth weight 4 lbs. or less—excluding those with cerebral palsy, blindness or deafness—the proportion of severely subnormal exceeded that expected in the normal population, being 18/1000 instead of about 3·7/1000. At 3 lbs. or less the proportion rose to 36/1000. Among singleton children weighing 4 lbs. or less at birth, with cerebral palsy, blindness or deafness, the proportion who were severely subnormal rose to 144/1000. Of all children (twins and singleton) under 4 lbs. (including blind, deaf and cerebral palsied) 26/1000 scored IQs of under 50. Because low birth weight is more common among lower social class births (Baird 1962)[2] this is one possible cause of the excess of severely subnormal subjects among children of lower social class families. It is unlikely in this country to be a numerically important cause of severe subnormality because only 7/1000 of all live births weigh less than 3 lbs. 4 oz. and just over one-third of these (344/1000 in 1962) survive for 28 days (Ministry of Health, 1963)*.

As Dr Fraser Roberts suggests, in the category of very low birth weight associated with severe subnormality, it is not clear whether the low birth weight causes the abnormality or whether the abnormality arises independently and causes the low birth weight. In considering the contribution of low birth weight to low intelligence I think it is useful to examine the two grades of subnormality (severe and mild) and the two ranges of birth weight (4–5½ lbs. and under 4 lbs.) separately. While this is helpful when looking at large numbers of cases, I am sure that the problem of individual cases which confronts the clinician is much more difficult.

REFERENCES

1. Åkesson, H. O. 1961. *Epidemiology and Genetics of Mental Deficiency in a Southern Swedish Population.* Uppsala. University of Uppsala.

* 1963. Ministry of Health of the State of Public Health. The Annual Report of the Chief Medical Officer of the Ministry of Health for the Year 1962. London. H.M.S.O.

2. BAIRD, D. 1962. Environmental and obstetrical factors in prematurity with special reference to experience in Aberdeen. *Bull. Wld. Hlth. Org.* **26**, 291–295.
3. BERG, J. M. and KIRMAN, B. H. 1959. Some aetiological problems in mental deficiency. *Brit. med. J.* ii, 848–852.
4. BUTLER, N. R. and BANHAM, D. G. 1963. *Perinatal Mortality.* London and Edinburgh. Livingstone.
5. CLARKE, A. D. B. and CLARKE, A. M. 1954. Cognitive changes in the feebleminded. *Brit. J. Psychol.* **45**, 173–179.
6. CLARKE, A. D. B., CLARKE, A. M. and REIMAN, S. 1958. Cognitive and social changes in the feebleminded ; three further studies. *Brit. J. Psychol.* **49**, 144–157.
7. COSER, ROSE L. 1962. *Life in the Ward.* East Lansing, Michigan. Michigan State University Press.
8. CROME, L. 1960. The brain and mental retardation. *Brit. med. J.* i, 879–904.
9. CRUICKSHANK, R. 1958. A survey of respiratory illnesses in a sample of families in London. In *Recent Studies in Epidemiology.* (Ed. J. Pemberton and H. Willard.) Oxford.
10. DOUGLAS, J. W. B. and BLOMFIELD, J. M. 1958. *Children under Five.* London. Allen and Unwin.
11. DUNSDON, M. I., CARTER, C. O. and HUNTLEY, R. M. C. 1960. Upper end of range of intelligence in mongolism. *Lancet* i, 565–568.
12. FARQUAR, J. W., RICHMOND, J. and TAIT, H. P. 1963. Phenylketonuria in pediatric practice: A review. *Clin. Pediat.* **2**, 504–516.
13. GOFFMAN, E. 1957. *The Characteristics of the Total Institution.* Walter Reed Symposium on Social Psychiatry. Washington, D.C.
14. GOODMAN, N. and TIZARD, J. 1962. Prevalence of imbecility and idiocy among children. *Brit. med. J.* i, 216–219.
15. GRAD, JACQUELINE and SAINSBURY, P. 1963. Mental illness and the family. *Lancet* i, 544–597.
16. HEADY, J. A., STEVENS, C. F., DALY, C. and MORRIS, J. N. 1955. Social and biological factors in infant mortality. IV. The independent effects of social class, region, the mother's age and her parity. *Lancet* i, 499–502.
17. *The Health of the School Child, 1960 and 1961.* 1962. Report of the Chief Medical Officer of the Ministry of Education. London. H.M.S.O.
18. *Health and Welfare: The Development of Community Care.* (Cmd. 1937.) 1963. London. H.M.S.O.
19. HILLIARD, L. T. and KIRMAN, B. H. 1965. *Mental Deficiency.* London. Churchill.
20. ILLINGWORTH, R. S. 1961. The predictive value of developmental tests in the first year with special reference to the diagnosis of mental subnormality. *J. Child Psychol. Psychiat.* **2**, 210–215.

21. KUSHLICK, A. 1961. Subnormality in Salford. In Susser, M. W. and Kushlick, A. *A Report on the Mental Health Services of the City of Salford for the Year 1960* pp. 18–48. Salford Health Department.

22. KUSHLICK, A. 1964. Prevalence of recognized mental subnormality of I.Q. under 50 among children in the south of England with reference to the demand for places for residential care. Paper to the *International Copenhagen Conference on the Scientific Study of Mental Retardation, Copenhagen, August* 1964.

23. KUSHLICK, A. 1965. Community care for the subnormal—a plan for evaluation. *Proc. roy. Soc. Med.* **58**, 374–380.

23*a*. KUSHLICK, A. Social problems in mental subnormality. In *The Foundation of Child Psychiatry.* (Ed. E. Miller) Oxford. Pergamon. In press.

24. LEESON, J. 1960. A study of six mentally handicapped children and their families. *Medical Officer* **104**, 311.

25. LEMKAU, P., TIETZE, C. and COOPER, M. 1942. Mental hygiene problems in an urban district. Third paper. *Mental Hygiene* **26**, 275-288.

26. LEWIS, E. O. 1929. *The Report of the Mental Deficiency Committee Being a Joint Committee of the Board of Education and Board of Control: Part IV—Report on an investigation into the incidence of mental deficiency in six areas,* 1925–1927. London. H.M.S.O.

27. LYLE, J. G. The effect of an institution environment upon the verbal development of imbecile children:
1959. Verbal intelligence. *J. ment. Defic. Res.* **3**, 122–128.

28. 1960*a*. Speech and language. *J. ment, Defic. Res.* **4**, 1–13.

29. 1960*b*. The Brooklands residential family unit. *J. ment. Defic. Res.* **4**, 14–23.

30. MENTAL HEALTH RESEARCH UNIT: Technical Report. 1955. *A Special Census of Suspected Referred Mental Retardation.*

31. MINISTRY OF EDUCATION. 1963. *Half our Future.* A report of the Central Advisory Council for Education (England). London. H.M.S.O.

32. MINISTRY OF HEALTH. 1964. *The Health and Welfare Services: Report for the Year ended* 31*st December* 1963. (Cmnd. 2389). London. H.M.S.O.

33. PARSONS, T. and BALES, R. F. 1955. *Family Socialization and Interaction Process.* Glencoe, Illinois. Free Press.

34. PENROSE, L. S. 1963. *The Biology of Mental Defect.* 3rd ed. London. Sidgwick and Jackson.

35. REGISTRAR GENERAL. 1958. *Decennial Supplement, England and Wales,* 1951. *Occupation Mortality, Part II: Civil.* London. H.M.S.O.

36. REGISTRAR GENERAL. 1960. *Statistical Review of England and Wales for the three years* 1954–1956. Supplement on Mental Health. London. H.M.S.O.

37. REGISTRAR GENERAL. 1961. *Statistical Review of England and Wales for the two years* 1957–1958. Supplement on Mental Health. London. H.M.S.O.

38. Registrar General. 1964. *Statistical Review of England and Wales for the year* 1960. Supplement on Mental Health. London. H.M.S.O.
39. Scottish Council for Research in Education. 1953. *Social Implications of the* 1947 *Scottish Mental Survey XXXV*. London. University of London Press.
40. Shotwell, Anna M. and Shipe, Dorothy. 1964. Effect of out-of-home care on the intellectual and social development of mongoloid children. *Amer. J. ment. Defic.* **68**, 693–699.
41. Stein, Zena and Susser, Mervin, M. W.
1960*a* Families of dull children:
Part II. Identifying family types and subcultures.
Part III. Social selection by family type.
Part IV. Increments in intelligence.
J. ment. Sci. **106**, 1296–1319.
1960*b* The families of dull children. A classification for predicting careers.
Brit. J. prev. soc. Med. **14**, 83–88.
42. Stein, Zena and Susser, Mervin, M. W. 1963. The social distribution of mental retardation. *Amer. J. ment. Defic.* **67**, 811–821.
43. Subnormality, Report of the Working Party. 1963. *Bull. Brit. psychol. Soc.* **16**, 37–50.
44. Tizard, J. 1958. Longitudinal and follow-up studies. In *Mental Deficiency—The Changing Outlook*. (Eds. A. M. and A. D. B. Clarke). London. Oxford University Press.
45. Tizard, J. and Grad, J. C. 1961. *The Mentally Handicapped and Their Families*. London. Oxford University Press.
46. Tizard, J. 1964. *Community Services for the Mentally Handicapped*. London. Oxford University Press.

BIOCHEMICAL ASPECTS OF MENTAL SUBNORMALITY *

C. E. Dent

University College Hospital Medical School, London

THE study of biochemical abnormalities as a cause of human disease is a very important subject of theoretical as well as of practical interest, especially as it so particularly involves the problem of mental subnormality, this awful dump of human misery which has been so largely neglected in the past by the academic research worker. I shall here try to generalize and bring out what is being learnt about the mechanisms by which

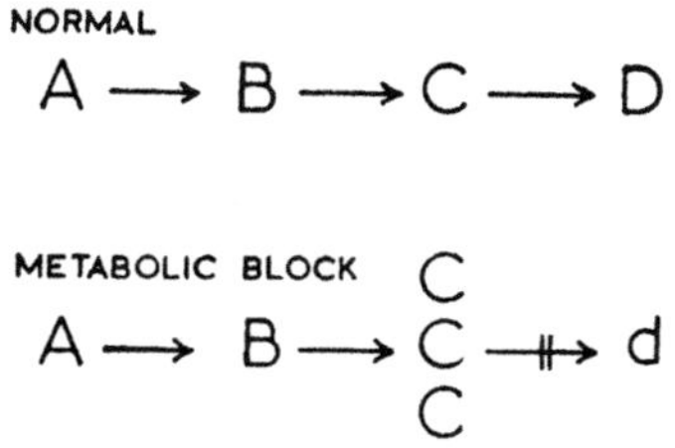

FIGURE 1

MECHANISM OF METABOLIC BLOCK

Metabolites are shown as letters, appropriate enzymes by arrows.

some biochemical abnormalities damage the brain. I shall try to describe a few general principles concerning these mechanisms, and in particular how we may hope to be able to modify them when discovered, and to show how far we have actually got with treatment, because, of course, it is painfully obvious that some of our work is purely observational, with no hope at the moment of useful treatment. Fortunately, however, there are some happy exceptions.

Figure 1 summarizes the simple diagram for which we have to thank Garrod who, fifty years ago, coined the term 'inborn error of metabolism'. It shows the mechanism of a particular kind of metabolic abnormality. Let us assume that in the

* An edited transcript of the verbatim report of Professor Dent's contribution to the Symposium.

course of normal metabolism the primary product is A, intermediary products are B and C, and the end product is D, probably excreted in the urine. Garrod's view was that in certain abnormalities—inborn errors—one of the enzymes shown by arrows is missing. If it is the arrow after C, it is obvious that there will be accumulation of the substance before, namely C, and an absence of the substance afterwards, D. This diagram represents, but in biochemical terms, a sort of mass production factory in which, so to speak, at each stage when one chemical compound is turned into another an enzyme is present which may be compared with a piece of machinery in the production line, or with a man using his hands. Stage by stage in the factory a piece of metal gradually turns into a motor car. It is the same with these biochemical mechanisms. The enzyme—the biochemical piece of machinery—is, like the machine, a highly specific and very complex substance and very often can do only one, usually simple, thing—turn B into C or C into D ; and obviously if one of the biochemical machines breaks down, accumulation of the immediate precursor is likely to occur. Then embarrassment is caused to the management, as to the human body, either because it is an infernal nuisance to have too much of C or because there is too little of D. In the factory they want the end product, and it is the absent motor car which is going to make the firm bankrupt. Ideally, the method of treatment would be to replace the damaged machine by another similar one or to try in some other way to substitute for the defect. It is clear now that in the medical application, with the corresponding biochemical disorder, D, the end product, which is something we are throwing away, does not matter so much as does the motor car in the factory. Very few diseases—one of these is albinism—are due to the absence of the end product, in this case the pigment in the skin. More usually the trouble is that the substance which accumulates, C, is 'toxic' using the word in its most general meaning, namely damaging by too much of it being present. The degree of abnormality, measured in terms of blood levels, is perhaps twenty or thirty times normal. This damages tissue growth, so that treatment must be directed to the artificial decrease

L

of C, either by increasing its excretion or by lessening its formation.

How does this damage the tissues and why does this kind of disordered mechanism produce so many specific and widely different forms of disease? One would like to think that this genetic abnormality would have to be present in all cells, having arisen from one cell in the first place at conception. However, with the specialization of tissues which occurs during normal growth, certain cells may manifest the abnormality more than others and the enzyme in question may appear to affect, shall we say, only the brain or liver. Thus it is possible to consider the medical condition as being localized, with the abnormality in only one part of the body.

The next point I want to make is illustrated in Figure 2. Suppose that normally tissue A is present in, say, intestinal mucous membrane, and forms sugars and amino acids from the diet, then releasing them into the body's extra-cellular fluid so as to bathe the other tissues of the body. Let us assume that tissue B is nutritionally dependent upon tissue A for some compound that thus reaches it via the blood and circulatory system. If there is something wrong with tissue A leading to an accumulation of the metabolite x from the type of disorder shown in Figure 1, all other functions being normal, two things can happen. In the first place, this substance x may be of large molecular weight—e.g, glycogen—in which case it will stay inside the cell and accumulate there. If it is harmful it will damage the particular organ which is making it, but no other organ. The extra-cellular fluid will not show any particular changes and other tissues will not be affected. We are in trouble at once with this kind of disorder, not knowing what to do about correcting the defect which seems so inaccesible to us. There are, unfortunately, many diseases of this kind, usually described as 'storage diseases'. Another difficulty is that, as already stated, all inborn errors (as well as most of our normal physical characteristics) are determined at the moment of conception though they may not begin to manifest the disease signs until tissue differentiation takes place within the next few months. But, since these errors are prenatal, some damage must be done *in utero* and is therefore obviously very difficult to prevent. In the present state of knowledge it is virtually impossible to speculate about how we could deal with this sort of abnormality.

Another situation is that shown on the right of Figure 2. It is one which admits of more hope and can at once consider as potentially curable. Here the substance accumulated is represented in the Figure as y instead of x. In this case the substance is assumed to be of small molecular weight and

Normal	IEM of Tissue A which overproduces non-diffusible metabolite x	IEM of Tissue A which overproduces diffusible metabolite y
(*a*)	(*b*)	(*c*)

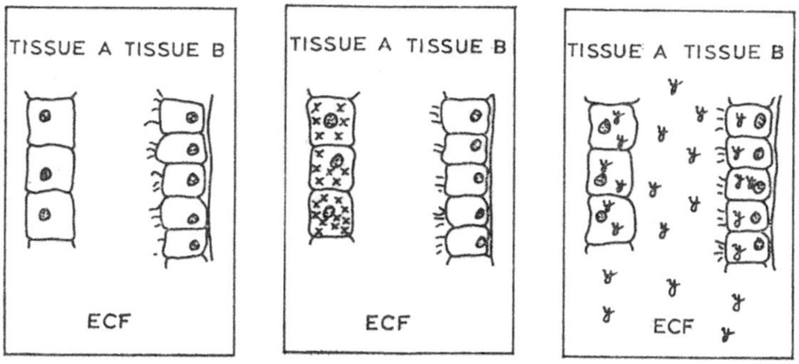

	A	B	A	B
Result of IEM	May be damaged	Normal	May be damaged	May be damaged
Dating of tissue damage	May be before birth	—	May be before birth	After birth
Therapeutic measures	Impossible in present state of knowledge		Possible	Possible

FIGURE 2

MECHANISMS OF TISSUE DAMAGE

(*a*) Normal. (*b*) Tissue A accumulates blocked metabolite x which may or may not damage tissue A but can have no effect elsewhere. (*c*) Tissue A forms excessive quantities of blocked metabolite y which diffuses into body fluids and is therefore less likely to damage tissue A but may damage tissue B if this more sensitive.

therefore able to pass through the cell membrane more easily. It will therefore get out of the cell where it was being produced, into the body fluid. Our problem then is whether we can get rid of it ; but it may, while circulating in the blood, thereby damage another tissue. Therapeutic measures are possible here because the disordered process is more accessible to investigation ; the compound can be found in easily obtainable body fluids (blood, urine), analysed quantitively, and measures for getting rid of it can be considered and their efficacy checked. A further important point must be made here: the damage from a readily diffusible small molecule is very likely to begin only after birth, after one has the baby in one's hands. The reason is, of course, that a diffusible substance of this kind formed by the baby is likely to be excreted through the placenta into the mother's blood, and she almost certainly has adequate biochemical machinery for destroying it. This certainly has been proved to happen in some metabolic disorders. The mother thus protects the child *in utero* and the damage does not start until after the child is born and has to rely on itself alone. Therapy in this sort of disordered biochemical mechanism is at once feasible in a variety of ways.

Another reason why this second type of disorder is much more likely to be amenable to treatment than the first is, of course, that we know much more about the chemistry of small diffusible molecules ; the biochemist has often worked it all out for us in advance and we can at once start thinking about what the details of the disorder are, and how to correct it. On the other hand, if we are dealing with large complicated molecules such as muco-saccharides, cerebrosides and such like, we are in difficulty, because the chemistry is not adequately known ; we hardly know any details of their structure, much less of how they are formed.

Another general principle is that the degree of damage to a tissue, and whether or not it occurs at all owing to the accumulation of a particular toxic metabolite, depends upon the rate of growth of that particular tissue, which can vary considerably with age. Figure 3 shows diagrammatically a simple scheme illustrating growth in rats and what happens if it is interfered with. Working with matched white rats is like working with little bits of precision machinery; they all grow at almost exactly the same speed if they are all fed in the same way. If for any reason—and the lines across the diagram represent some sort of insult to the animal—the diet is adversely changed, some vitamin left out or the diet made inadequate in any other way, growth slows or stops for as long as the insult is continued. Then, if the rat is put again on a normal diet, it will grow faster for a time and, depending upon how long the inadequate

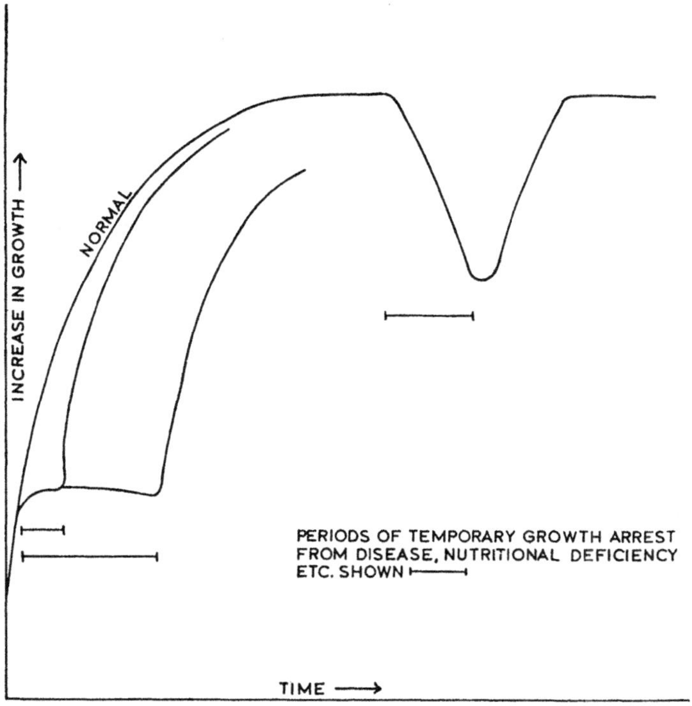

FIGURE 3

HYPOTHETICAL RAT GROWTH CURVES, NORMAL AND WHEN AFFECTED ADVERSELY BY SOME DIETARY OR OTHER INADEQUACY FOR THE DURATION OF THE HORIZONTAL LINE

Similar curves apply to the growth of single organs or tissues but the time scale will be widely different.

diet has lasted, its weight will or will not get nearer and nearer to the original growth line ; so it will probably end up almost as big as if the check had not happened, though when the check has lasted a long time, the adult ends up as a small rat. This latter is what we see, I am sure, with different peoples who have not been fed adequately in childhood ; even in Britain we see the difference between Scotland and London, with 5 ft. 1 in. mothers in Dundee, as Professor Walker has just shown. Once people have reached adult size, of course, they are far less sensitive to these influences. Those of us who have seen unfortunate concentration-camp victims know that, if a person who has once reached adult size is starved and becomes a scarecrow for a time but does not suffer some accident as a result of the starvation (which often predisposes to tuberculosis, dysentery and death from other causes) but is rescued and re-fed, he ends up almost exactly the same as he was before. I have shown this on the graph ; one can temporarily inhibit an adult person, but he is far less sensitive to permanent growth damage than the growing child ; which of course is the very good reason why rationing in war-time was made more liberal for children.

This refers not only to whole animals but also to particular tissues. We should be especially interested in the brain, the organ which grows fastest of all immediately after birth ; it grows faster for a time than any tumour but rapidly slows down afterwards. If any metabolic defect is present soon after birth, it is very likely to damage the brain, even if it does not appreciably damage the whole body or any other tissues at the same time. Likewise, at different ages other tissues may be affected more than the brain, which reaches adult size long before any other organ and can then be insulted with comparative impunity. These points are very relevant in studying the clinical manifestation of a biochemical defect.

Let us now illustrate these general mechanisms by mentioning in more detail four of these diseases. The first one I will deal with is a terrible, acute disorder of the neonatal period, the so-called ‘ maple syrup urine ’ disease from which children often die at the eighth day of life, or more often when about a month old ; they hardly ever survive longer, but if they do, they are all severely brain-damaged. They are all, as far as we know, absolutely normal at birth ; it is the second mechanism, with the diffusible metabolite *y* in Figure 2, that is operative in these cases.

The chemistry involves the three aliphatic amino acids which are unique in possessing branched carbon chains (leucine, isoleucine and valine). It is called maple syrup urine disease because of the smell of the urine in the untreated state. It is the accumulation of these amino acids and break-down products of metabolism that damages the child. We were fortunate to be responsible for a new-born infant whose mother had had a previous affected child, and who gave birth to the new child in our hospital. This new child appeared quite normal at birth. The cord blood was obtained and was normal. The amino acids and everything else were normal, but nevertheless we watched to see what would happen. In the next few days the characteristic abnormalities appeared in the blood and urine and it became obvious that here was another case of maple syrup urine disease. Fortunately, the placenta had done its unaccustomed job of preventing any permanent accumulation of the metabolites until the time the child was born, and therefore there were strong biochemical reasons, as well as clinical ones, for expecting the child to be quite normal at that time.

Chromatograms of blood and urine of the first days of the baby's life illustrate graphically exactly how the abnormalities were developing in this child in the first five days of its life, the cord blood being at first absolutely normal and then going wrong because, for dietary reasons, the amino acids were being supplied in excess and the child could not destroy the extra. On the fifth day the child started to vomit and go off its food. We already had the biochemical evidence and were able to put the child on a diet restricting the quantity of these metabolites so as to make this plasma more normal. Then, after about another four days, everything went back to normal: we were producing artificially by diet the same state as the baby had been in *in utero* when the mother was doing the job for it via the placenta. This is the sort of disease where measuring results of treatment presents no problem ; it is such a grossly abnormal condition that there is no need for control experiments. One can tell what is happening just by looking at the child, and nobody could suggest that there was some other interpretation of its response to the diet than the one we have given.

At two years of age the child showed absolutely normal development after continuing on a diet of special food supplied in cartons and bottles to the mother every two-to-three weeks. The mother adds water to the powders to make up the volume and the child takes it without hesitation. As to the economics, the raw material price of this special diet is about 15s. a day, paid as a matter of routine by the NHS. At the age of four the child is still perfectly normal, physically and mentally.

I hesitate to mention this, but here we are, by saving these children's lives, encouraging these unfortunate, unpleasant genes to continue and reproduce themselves in the population as a whole. We do this shamelessly, even proudly. I can only say it is awfully nice of the Eugenics Society to invite me to contribute to this Symposium.

The next disease I will discuss is phenylketonuria. The chemical abnormality in the blood is readily demonstrated on a paper chromatogram developed to show the amino acid composition. It comprises a large spot for the amino acid phenylalanine, instead of the normal smaller one. Quantitative analysis shows the abnormality to be about 20 times normal. All the other constituents, however, are normal. It is interesting to contemplate how simple and specific this analysis is in the presence of a clinical picture which is not very specific, and one which had never been distinguished in any way from other forms of mental deficiency, until the chemistry was first defined. We know now that the blood of the affected baby, as in maple syrup urine disease, is normal at birth. The abnormality develops in the next few days but is not so acutely harmful as in MSU disease ; so the brain damage develops more slowly over the next few months. Nevertheless, the sooner it is diagnosed and treated the better, the principles of treatment being the same as in MSU disease. There is a great difficulty here in assessing the results of treatment since inevitably the effects of treatment in preventing the brain damage from occurring are also slower to manifest themselves. This led originally to some controversy among the original workers as to its efficacy. An important study by Woolf, Griffiths and others, shown in Figure 3, illustrates the time scale of the disease with and without treatment and has produced curves for mental development rather similar to those shown diagrammatically for body growth in rats in Figure 1. The study shows first that the fall in mental age of untreated phenylketonurics, compared with normal, is greater the older the child is ; in other words, progressive slow brain damage has been occurring. Secondly, from the time that treatment by diet is begun, the rate of development of mental age increases (arrow A) at at least a normal rate. The diet, however, was, and still is, a difficult one to keep to and many mothers defaulted for one reason or another. When this happened (arrow B) the increase of mental age with chronological age decreased in rate, to increase again (arrow C) when, on discovery of the situation, more pressure was brought to bear on the mothers to be meticulous with the diet.

Obviously one of the important things is this question of how soon treatment is started. The problem of how long it has to go on (as yet unsettled) depends also on factors of that kind. Another point is that if something goes wrong with the diet for a very short time, not very much damage happens to a phenylketonuric child, a more fortunate situation than in maple syrup urine disease, but one which may, however, occasionally tempt the mother to stop the diet altogether. In contrast, with maple syrup urine disease, transgressions in the diet, and other circumstances that can make the child ill, may be so slight that we have not always been able to discover what has actually gone wrong, although we had no doubt from the analysis that it must have been due to environmental factors.

Another disease upon which we have been working, homocystinuria, is one in which the time scale of events is even more prolonged. Dietary protein breaks down in the gut to the amino acids, one of which is methionine. It is interesting that in the metabolic sequence in the subsequent breakdown

CORRIGENDUM

Page 157, line 5. Delete " shown in Figure 3 "

of methionine in the tissues, two abnormalities have been discovered, both of which produce mental deficiency: cystathioninuria and homocystinuria, the latter comprising a block in metabolism in which homocystine accumulates in the tissues, blood and urine. The course of events in the latter disease is even slower than it is in phenylketonuria ; in fact we strongly suspect that these children are almost normal for the first few years of life. In one of our cases, a boy who came to us at the age of fifteen, we were able to get photographs of him taken earlier in life. They showed that at the age of two-and-a-half he certainly *looked* normal. A few months later he still looked quite normal. When he later went to school, he did not do too well and the parents were advised to send him to a special school. For some years they refused to accept this opinion and paid for him to go to an ordinary private school. It was some while before they would accept their doctor's opinion that he was somewhat retarded. The photograph of him at six years of age showed that he was developing knock-knee and spindly legs ; his eyesight was deteriorating ; yet his abnormality still had not fully developed. When he presented himself to us at the age of fifteen years he had very long spindly legs and gross knock-knees which had recurred following their straightening by osteotomy a couple of years before. By now he was almost blind owing to grossly dislocated lenses. Here we see a much longer time scale, much less acute than the others. At the age of fifteen years he was not so mentally retarded as would be the average phenylketonuric, because his brain was not damaged so soon after birth, when it is so much more sensitive. The toxic process was present then, but was having a much milder action. Just as would be expected in this sort of delayed onset disease, we are noting, now that it is being identified more and more, that the mental retardation and the other signs of disease that slowly develop are exceedingly variable in degree from one case to another. In fact, some cases are being found with fairly normal IQ in adult life presumably because of some dietary peculiarity which lessened the degree of biochemical abnormality in the first ten to twenty years of life. This is where environment comes into the situation more and more and the genetic effect is less prominent, a situation more familiar to us in our well-known infectious diseases. Older homocystinuric patients with their long limbs and eye abnormality look superficially like cases of Marfan's syndrome (arachnodactyly) and have obviously been confused with these latter in the past. McKusick has recently shown that about 5 per cent of his large series of patients with alleged Marfan's syndrome were indeed suffering from homocystinuria. It appears that homocystinuria is a relatively common cause of mental retardation—about half as common as phenylketonuria on first estimate. Most of the other known biochemical causes of mental deficiency are much rarer than this.

The fourth disease I will mention briefly, Wilson's disease, illustrates an even more slowly developing disease process due to an inborn error of metabolism. Perhaps it is for this reason that the higher brain centres are hardly damaged at all. In Wilson's disease we see a clear instance of the environment influencing the actual genetic disorder because it is very much concerned with copper metabolism and inability to protect the body against the ordinary dietary intake of copper. Although it is still pure speculation, the evidence strongly suggests that the age of onset of the disease depends upon how much copper the person has eaten. Likewise, the ensuing clinical features of the disease depend upon the age of onset. Wilson's disease patients, if they grow ill in childhood, mainly show symptoms related to cirrhosis of the liver. I think the reason is that at that stage the liver is growing faster than any other organ and is therefore more sensitive. Later in life other organs, such as the kidneys, get damaged by Wilson's disease. We see a great variation in clinical pictures with such a late onset disease, which our biochemical theory forces us also to attribute to the varying environment. It is important to emphasize that this situation gives us much greater scope for more simple treatment, since some natural environmental conditions are here clearly consistent with normal health, even in the presence of the inborn error. In the case of Wilson's disease the evidence indicating that most of the disease manifestations are due to poisoning by the normal copper content of the diet is supported by the results of treatment. Drugs such as penicillamine, which can cause a degree of copper depletion, can cure most of the disease manifestations even when given to rather well-established cases and in spite of the fact that no more fundamental attempt to correct the inborn enzyme defect is made, as is necessary in the cases mentioned before.

Everything I have said about inborn errors concerned with specific deficiencies of enzymes may also be mimicked by diseases of environmental origin. Some toxins such as lead or phthalidomide, or some deficiencies such as of vitamins or of atmospheric oxygen, can damage specifically many tissues and enzymic processes at the same time ; which makes it rather difficult to give a biochemical interpretation. On the other hand, drugs are known now which can damage single enzymes and thus mimic very closely the very specific metabolic disorder which some people inherit. Really there is no particular difference in principle between acquired and environmental conditions ; they may resemble each other closely, and we must never be defeatist and imagine that an inherited disorder is some sort of hopeless, miserable curse. The same general principles apply to environmental disease, in that the damage depends on age and on rate of growth ; and which particular body organ is involved in any particular case very much depends on the nature and rate of metabolism of that organ and on the state at which it differentiates in the embryo. We have therefore also in mainly environmental diseases severe and more homogeneous manifestations and usually brain damage, when they do their damage to the very young baby, but when the disease is milder and more delayed the manifestations are less homogeneous.

In summary we must emphasize that we still are left with many diseases which we cannot now treat or even speculate how in the future we may be able to treat, because the substances formed are intra-cellular and do not diffuse into the body fluids (x in Figure 2). Then we have a whole host of new ones, all obviously at sight amenable to treatment (y in Figure 2) though the details may not yet be worked out. Just as the placenta has protected the unborn child from these latter abnormalities of diffusible substances, so artificial ‘ placentas ’ should be able to do something in later life to protect people whom we cannot deal with in other ways. I have in mind here especially organs like the artificial kidney ; for we already know that, if a person has an abnormality in the blood due to acute kidney or liver disease, it is possible sometimes to help such people greatly by washing them out on an artificial kidney, a procedure which is becoming now quite easy to perform. I have already twice tried (alas unsuccessfully) using an artificial kidney on people who were severely mentally ill, to see if one does wash anything out and make them better, on the theory that their illness might be due to the presence of an as yet unidentified substance in their blood which I had hoped would be freely diffusible. I would recommend further trials of this sort as an alternative to a study of diseases in which the biochemical abnormality has already been discovered by other means. If we can make such people better with an artificial kidney, then of course the stuff we wash out is in the bath water and we can find and, I hope, identify it.

DISCUSSION

Professor Dent, when asked whether he himself had done any chromatograms on pregnant women where metabolic disorders were expected, and if the increase of amino acid was enough in comparison with the mother's secretion to show at that stage, replied that the one for maple syrup disease had been done very carefully and, as expected, it had not been found in the mother's urine though there might be findings in some of the other diseases in which the metabolite in question had a high renal clearance. One would expect to find it in such a mother's urine when she was carrying an abnormal baby, but tests for it had not yet been successful though the possibility had not been excluded.

Professor Dent agreed with another questioner that the task of testing all babies was an exacting one—in a large hospital the nurses carrying out the tests might discover the phenylketonuric baby once in five years—but he did not think that many were missed. From the doctor's point of view, as distinct from the research worker's, it was important to concentrate on the search for those abnormalities for which some treatment could be offered.

With regard to the little girl with maple syrup urine disease, the speaker was asked about the child's future prospects. He replied that she was too young for there to be a final answer ; she was now four years old, a lovely child, physically and mentally normal. It might be expected that she would grow out of it in a few years, because the pathology very much concerned myelin formation and damage to myelination. Once all the myelin had been formed, the child should be much more resistant to the biochemical abnormality. There was always the hope that better treatment might be discovered than that of using the complicated diet. The obvious way would be to increase the excretion of amino acids in the urine and enable the child to go on a normal diet. But these questions could not be answered yet. Though the mother was reasonably well adjusted, there were other family problems. In one case, although the child's food had been paid for under the NHS since birth (which had made it very cheap for the parents), the father had recently suggested that all clothing should also be supplied free !

BIBLIOGRAPHY FOR GENERAL READING

CARSON, N. A. J., DENT, C. E., FIELD, C. M. B. and GAULL, G. E. 1965. Homocystinuria: Clinical and pathological review. *J. Pediat.* **66**, 565.

DENT, C. E. 1957. General review of inborn errors of metabolism. *Amer. J. Med.* **22**, 671.

STANBURY, J. B., WYNGAARDEN, J. B. and FREDRICKSON, D. S. 1960. *Metabolic Basis of Inherited Disease.* London. McGraw-Hill.

WESTALL, R. G. 1963. Dietary treatment of a child with maple syrup urine disease. *Arch. Dis. Child.* **38**, 485.

WOOLF, L. I., GRIFFITHS, R., MONTCRIEFF, A., COATES, S. and DILLISTONE, F. 1958. Dietary treatment of phenylketonuria. *Arch. Dis. Child.* **33**, 31.

CHROMOSOMAL ASPECTS OF MENTAL SUBNORMALITY

VALERIE COWIE

MRC Psychiatric Genetics Research Unit, Maudsley Hospital, S.E. 5, *and Queen Mary's Hospital for Children, Carshalton, Surrey*

DURING the past few years there has been a marked shift of interest in human genetics towards a direct study of the cell as a replicating unit. This has been made possible mainly by a breakthrough in cytogenetical techniques. We are still concerned with deductions in genetics that can be made from the distribution of traits in populations and in families ; but the recent advances have added a new dimension and brought us closer to the chromosomes and their substance, which is the stuff of heredity itself. In the study of human genetics within the cell, there is still scope for further work at various levels. Thus a distinction can be drawn between problems which can be approached using techniques of chromosomal analysis, and others which lend themselves to biochemical investigation or statistical treatment. At our present stage of development chromosomal techniques are rewarding only when fairly major changes can be seen under the microscope. Biochemical methods on the other hand can probe deeper, indicating, for example, gene-enzyme relationships.

The advances in cytogenetics have been remarkable considering that before the reported observations of Tjio and Levan [20] in 1956 even the number of chromosomes in the human cell was in doubt. Our methods for preparing chromosomes for analysis have improved since that time, and although we have been working all along up to the limits of resolution—which have been advancing in step with technical progress—we have now perhaps reached an optimum for a rewarding observation of the number, size and morphology of the chromosomes. This is due only in part to technical limits. It is due mainly to the properties of the chromosomes themselves: to the size of the human chromosomes in tissues available for culture, and to the lack of landmarks upon them. Special techniques, such as the autoradiography of chromosomes cultured with a medium containing labelled thymidine, are being tried in an effort to identify individual chromosomes, but this problem of identification still exists, and often it is not possible even to identify pairs of chromosomes in a normal karyotype with certainty.

Despite these difficulties numerous findings have been made ; but in this field we are still very much at the stage of Gilbert White at Selborne. We are still collecting and recording our observations, and on the basis of our interpretations we are making attempts at classification. At present these attempts rely mainly on what we see in the chromosomal pattern and on clinical signs. They are still largely descriptive, therefore, and are connected with structure rather than with dynamics and function.

The time seems to have come when it would be profitable to stand back and make a fresh evaluation of the significance of chromosomal abnormalities in connection with the physical and psychological phenomena associated with them. It is all too easy to become like a stamp collector, and never look beyond the fascinating array before one's eyes. In this frame of mind it is comfortable to think of abnormalities in the chromosomal pattern as being of primary aetiological significance and to ascribe to them specific individual effects and constellations of signs. In this way one may be beguiled into forcing observations into a rigid classification, so that fresh thinking is discouraged and the collection becomes an end in itself.

AUTOSOMAL ANOMALIES AND MENTAL SUBNORMALITY

Cytogenetics is of special importance in connection with mental subnormality, because marked mental defect is an almost constant concomitant of autosomal anomalies, and mental impairment of milder degree is not infrequently found in the presence of sex chromosome anomalies. It is notable that mongolism was the first human condition to be found in association with an autosomal defect by Lejeune [12] and his co-workers in 1959. This is still the most famous and the most widely studied of the syndromes associated with a chromosomal anomaly, no doubt on account of its relatively high incidence in the general population, a mongol baby being born to one in probably less than every 666 mothers giving birth to live or stillborn children.[1, 21] The classically accepted chromosomal defect in mongolism is a triplication of a chromosome in the G group, the extra chromosome existing separately or a major part of it being fused to another in the form of a translocation. Other syndromes, less common than mongolism but exemplified by a number of reported cases have been described in association with specific autosomal defects. These include trisomy of a chromosome of the E group (first described by Edwards and his co-workers in 1960 [7]), trisomy of a chromosome of the D group (first described by Patau and his team, 1960 [17]) and the *cri-du-chat* syndrome described by Lejeune and his co-workers,[13] which is associated, not with extra chromosomal material, but with a deletion of part of a chromosome in the B group.

Besides the chromosomal defects associated with these syndromes, many anomalies involving other autosomes have been described. These, however—unlike the repeatedly recurring conditions such as mongolism—have been sporadic in incidence. But both with sporadic and with repeatedly observed examples of autosomal abnormalities, an outstanding and almost constant concomitant has been mental defect, often of profound degree. In many cases structural abnormalities have been found in the brain on neuropathological examination.

SEX CHROMOSOME ANOMALIES AND MENTAL SUBNORMALITY

Turning to abnormalities of the sex chromosomes, we find that, on the whole, the associated physical defects are milder than with autosomal anomalies, although there are often characteristically profound pathological changes in the gonads. In individuals with autosomal abnormalities it seems that all tissues in the body are affected, but with sex chromosome abnormalities the burden of defect seems to lie in the genital tract.[3] The frequency with which mental defect is associated with sex chromosome anomalies is open to question and a bias in favour of the association may have arisen through the number of sex-chromatin surveys that have been carried out in Institutions for the mentally subnormal. As Israelson and Taylor [10] pointed out, further studies are needed if the theory that cases of chromatin-positive Klinefelter's syndrome (as an example of the most prevalent type of sex chromosome anomaly) have their highest incidence in the borderline or low-normal intelligence range is to be maintained. Moreover, as these workers remark, psychometric studies on a larger number of chromatin-positive cases and their families are needed to provide evidence of the extent to which the brain can develop and function normally in the presence of an abnormal sex-chromosome complement.

It seems clear, however, that the degree of mental impairment, when it does occur in connection with abnormalities involving the sex chromosomes, is less than when it occurs with autosomal changes. On the other hand, there is evidence to suggest an increase of personality disorders amongst people with abnormalities of the sex-chromosomes. The manifestations described tend to be non-specific and variable. For example, Pasqualini and his co-workers [16] remark upon the schizoid traits liable to be seen amongst individuals with Klinefelter's syndrome. Nielsen [14] described a mental hospital's patients with Klinefelter's syndrome as characteristically immature, sensitive and showing little initiative. He considered that such individuals were especially sensitive to all forms of stress, and that consequently they might be expected to develop mainly affective mental disorders or to be classified as having character disorders. Kidd and his co-workers [11] report a greater intensity of impairment of interpersonal relationships and a greater degree of social withdrawal in triple-*x* patients as compared with a control group. It is difficult to speculate upon any likely relationship between the rather diffuse psychiatric changes described and anomalies of the sex chromosomes, but as times goes on and more observations are made, some aetiological connection may emerge, perhaps, for example, involving the sex hormones.

THE RELATIONSHIP OF CLINICAL SIGNS TO CHROMOSOMAL ABNORMALITIES

Taking a broad view of the phenotypical features that accompany chromosomal abnormalities, one is struck by the recurrence of clinical signs, not only within groups of individuals with similar chromosomal defects, but between groups with different kinds of defects affecting different chromosomes. This applies chiefly to the autosomes, with which the accompanying physical signs are more striking than with the sex chromosomes. Certain organs and regions of the body seem particularly vulnerable. These include the orbits and periorbital structures, the nasal bridge, the mouth and palate, the pinnae of the ears, the lower jaw, the neck, the hands and feet, and the viscera, notably the heart. Moreover, these parts are seen to be affected in characteristic and unusual ways. For example, changes in the orbital and periorbital structures often become manifest as an abnormal slant of the palpebral fissures and epicanthus ; the hands not infrequently show the striking sign of a single horizontal palmar crease ; the feet may be grotesquely deformed with 'rocker-bottom' soles and protruding heels.

Although these abnormalities are occasionally met with in people who have no demonstrable chromosomal defects, the recurrence of the same clinical signs, which are often bizarre, in patients with different kinds of autosomal abnormality is suggestive of a degree of non-specificity in their clinical concomitants. A simple explanation might be sought on quantitative grounds. For example, one could conjecture that the extra chromosomal material in a trisomy might correspond to an imbalance affecting the development of specifically vulnerable regions of the body irrespective of which chromosomes were involved. One might go on to suppose that the constellations of more specific clinical signs that differentiate the classical trisomies are determined by gene loci on the extra chromosomes. Such explanations based on a quantitative hypothesis are, however, inadequate and altogether too facile, because the same basic bizarre specific clinical signs are seen to accompany autosomal defects where the chromosomal material present in the cell is deficient, not excessive, in quantity.

As we are here concerned with chromosomal anomalies in connection with mental subnormality, I would like to discuss this quantitative effect further in connection with the brain. It is not surprising that the brain, which is the most complex organ in the body and consists of the most highly differentiated tissue, should be especially vulnerable in the course of its development. Again, however, a particular vulnerability is observed—no matter what kind of chromosomal change takes place, what quantity of chromosomal material is present in the cell, or which chromosomes are involved—in that the fore-brain and its adjacent structures seem to be especially prone to maldevelopment. Thus hypoplasia or agenesis of the corpus callosum is not infrequently seen in trisomy D (Norman[15] and in trisomy E (Edwards [6]). This gross and rather unusual brain lesion has been found, however, in association with chromosomal anomalies involving autosomes outside the groups D and E, in which too little rather than too much chromatin has been present in the cells examined. Thus agenesis of the corpus callosum was found subsequent to the report [5] of a baby with multiple congenital anomalies and an apparently balanced karyotype carrying a reciprocal D/F translocation. It was thought that the abnormalities in this baby could be related to a position effect of translocated fragments, or to a minute deletion of chromosomal material, or to a combination of these. From a quantitative point of view, therefore, this child probably had too little rather than too much chromosomal material in his cells.

To sum up, a number of basic, often bizarre, clinical signs are common to a range of chromosomal defects, involving autosomes of different groups and involving quantitative changes in both directions. This would suggest that a broader view should be taken than the conventional one that specific lesions of chromosomes in specific groups have a causal relationship with specific clinical and pathological changes. Apart from these common basic phenotypical changes, however, it seems likely that characteristic clinical features by which the classical autosomal syndromes are distinguished, may be related to such factors as changes in the specific gene loci present.

At this stage it would seem more profitable to examine the clinical and pathological similarities than the differences between individuals with chromosomal defects. This would alter our viewpoint and probably bring us nearer to finding the relationship between chromosomal anomalies and physical and psychological changes. I think we may eventually come to see a hierarchy of aetiological phenomena, in which chromosomal changes are only one step on the way towards the shaping of the individual. As Penrose [19] pointed out, referring to the example of aneuploidy in plants, the distortions to growth which can follow may simply be a question of water balance in the cells. A broad biological approach to investigate possible cellular changes accompanying chromosomal alterations would seem to be a most promising line to follow, with experimental studies into cellular changes which may precede chromosomal changes, as well as more observational studies of cells with chromosome anomalies that have already occurred.

THE NEED FOR A MULTIDIMENSIONAL APPROACH

At the same time, I feel that our investigation of the problems associated with human chromosomal anomalies would be greatly facilitated by a multidimensional approach, involving close collaboration between the cytogeneticist and cellular biologist, the embryologist, the clinician, the biochemist, the neuropathologist and the psychologist. It is valuable to pool all the facts, in order to see the place of each in the aetiological sequence and allow the emergence of factors that might otherwise remain hidden. On account of the gene-enzyme relationship it is likely that the biochemist may be especially able to help in the intensely complex problem of how chromosomes influence not only growth and development but function. This might well have special implications for mental subnormality. On the whole, biochemical studies in mongolism have been disappointing, but we should not be put off by this ; it would be worthwhile to continue them and to make a systematic study of other conditions associated with chromosomal anomalies.

Moreover, we should not confine our biochemical and other studies exclusively to the individuals with demonstrable chromosome anomalies ; investigation of their relatives is also necessary. For instance, many years ago Penrose [18] suggested that an unusually high proportion of the relatives of mongols show ' microsymptoms ' of the condition. From time to time additional evidence [8, 9] has appeared supporting this suggestion, and there are indications of constitutional differences in mothers who have given birth at an early age to mongols.[2] Along these lines there is need of further work which may give a clue to genetical and constitutional factors predisposing to the occurrence of chromosomal abnormalities.

The study of relatives can be of very special significance in cytogenetics for another reason. The problem of identifying individual chromosomes was mentioned earlier. One of our handicaps in classifying chromosomal abnormalities results directly from this. We rely essentially on the size and number of the chromosomes for interpretation of the karyotype, unless a carrier is available. Carriers usually have a quantitatively balanced chromosomal complement, but the disposition of the components is altered, so that it is possible to track down the changes that have occurred. For example, a baby with mongolism, whom we examined recently, appeared to show a G/G translocation, which is an established variant in the condition. This would have been our interpretation had we not examined her father's chromosomes. We discovered that he carried an F/G translocation. From this the interpretation was made that in the baby's case the extra chromosomal material was derived from an F- rather than a G-group chromosome.[4] If we are right in this interpretation, the findings show that mongolism can exist without trisomy G.

Family studies may therefore yield information of special significance. For this reason, advancement in human cytogenetics calls for team-work. Without family data and careful and accurate clinical observations a great deal of vital information can be lost. Through necessity and tradition, there is already much good team-work among those working in the field of mental subnormality. This is particularly fortunate for those concerned with the study of human chromosomal abnormalities. At the same time, advancement in cytogenetics has done a great deal to draw attention to the potentialities for research into mental defect. On account of the close association between chromosomal anomalies and mental subnormality, the intellectually handicapped are of special significance in human biology. Again, to quote Penrose,[19] the mentally subnormal provide us with an unrivalled opportunity for examining the mode of evolution of the human race.

ACKNOWLEDGEMENTS

I am especially indebted to Dr Jacob Kahn of the MRC Psychiatric Genetics Unit, with whom many of the ideas discussed in this paper were developed, and to Dr Eliot Slater for his helpful advice and criticism.

REFERENCES

1. Carter, C. O. and MacCarthy, D. 1951. Incidence of mongolism and its diagnosis in the newborn. *Brit. J. soc. Med.* **5**, 83–90.
2. Coppen, A. and Cowie, V. 1960. Maternal health and mongolism. *Brit. med. J.* i, 1843–1847.
3. Court Brown, W. M. 1962. In *Cytogenetics in Medicine. R.C.P.E.*, No. 18.
4. Cowie, V. and Kahn, J. 1965. A mongol child without trisomy G. *Lancet* ii, 58–59.
5. Cowie, V., Kahn, J. and O'Reilly, J. N. 1965. Congenital abnormalities in a child with an apparently balanced karyotype carrying a reciprocal D/F translocation. *Lancet* i, 1043–1044.
6. Edwards, J. H. 1963. Personal communication.
7. Edwards, J. H., Harnden, D. G., Cameron, A. H., Crosse, V. M. and Wolff, O. H. 1960. A new trisomic syndrome. *Lancet* i, 787–790.
8. Fang, T. C. 1950. The third interdigital patterns on the palms of the general British population, mongoloid and non-mongoloid mental defectives. *J. ment. Sci.* **96**, 780–787.
9. Glanville, E. V. 1964. Mongolism: a clue to the source of the accessory chromosome? *Lancet* ii, 1065–1066.
10. Israelson, W. J. and Taylor, A. I. 1961. Chromatin-positive presumed Klinefelter's syndrome. *Brit. med. J.* i, 633–635.

11. Kidd, C. B., Knox, R. S. and Mantle, D. J. 1963. A psychiatric investigation of triple-x chromosome females. *Brit. J. Psychiat.* **109**, 90–94.

12. Lejeune, J., Gautier, M. and Turpin, R. 1959. Les chromosomes humains en culture de tissus. *C.R. Acad. Sci.* (*Paris*), **248**, 602–603.

13. Lejeune, J., Lafourcade, J., Berger, R., Vialatte, J., Boeswillwald, M., Seringe, P. and Turpin, R. 1963. Trois cas de délétion du bras court d'un chromosome 5. *C.R. Acad. Sci.*, (*Paris*), **257**, 3098–3102.

14. Nielsen, J. 1964. Prevalence of Klinefelter's syndrome in patients with mental disorders. (Letter to Editor.) *Lancet* i, 1109.

15. Norman, R. M. 1965. Personal communication.

16. Pasqualini, R. Q., Vidal, G. and Bur, G. E. 1957. Psychopathology of Klinefelter's syndrome. Review of thirty-one cases. *Lancet* ii, 164–167.

17. Patau, K., Smith, D. W., Therman, E., Inhorn, S. L. and Wagner, H. P. 1960. Multiple congenital anomaly caused by an extra chromosome. *Lancet* i, 790–793.

18. Penrose, L. S. 1954. The distal triradius *t* on the hands of parents and sibs of mongol imbeciles. *Ann. hum. Genet.* **19**, 10–38.

19. Penrose, L. S. 1962. Biological aspects. *Proc. Lond. Conf. Sci. Study ment. Def. July* 1960, i, 11–18.

20. Tjio, J. H. and Levan, A. 1956. Chromosome number in man. *Hereditas* **42**, 1–6.

21. Zappella, M. and Cowie, Valerie. 1962. A note on time of diagnosis in mongolism. *J. ment. Def. Res.* **6**, 82–86.

ASPECTS OF SUBNORMALITY

Conclusion

Brian H. Kirman
Queen Mary's Hospital for Children, Carshalton

I will not attempt to sum up this session. I think that would be a quite impossible task.

I do think it is most encouraging to see this assembly under these auspices. I would like to take up one point at which Professor Dent hinted: " What am I doing here ? " he almost said. I was asked that question also: why had I consented to take the chair in this connection, and was it not immoral ? What has happened, of course, is that over the past fifty years there has clearly been a very radical change in scientific outlook on this problem of mental retardation. If not the members of the Eugenics Society, then at least people interested in eugenics, perhaps amateur enthusiasts, early in the century were pontificating and making statements which have subsequently proved to be ill-founded. In contrast, to-day we have had very sophisticated papers presented, I should say, with an attitude of proper scientific humility, emphasizing both the questions awaiting answers and our present lack of knowledge. In spite of all that the speakers have told us, they have raised many more questions than they have answered ; they have indicated that we are just beginning to realize the importance of this field for the future of humanity.

At the same time, I think there has been a very considerable change in attitude, a change from pessimism and alarmism to cautious optimism. That too has emerged at this session. We do realize how extremely difficult this subject is to tackle both from the scientific and from the practical angle as regards doing something about it, but clearly we are optimistic now. There has been further change, in that we are no longer primarily concerned with single factors operating *in vacuo*, but do now understand a very little of the extremely delicate dialectics of this problem. We see the nice interrelationship of a large number of factors ; and those people who approach the problem from the point of view of comparative biology are also aware of the tremendous importance of social organization.

Dr Kushlick's contribution and the contributions of others have emphasized this. They have shown us that conclusions, which may have been true in conditions as they were fifty years ago, are not necessarily true where we have full employment and the provision of a large measure of social security. Thus, if the evolution of human society is developing—as it obviously is—much more rapidly than the evolution of the human individual at a biological level, we must take this fact very much into consideration in drawing conclusions as to what should be done in the way of social provision for the mentally retarded. From what has been said to-day it is clearly necessary that we should press for much more of this work to be done in view of its paramount importance. We must ask for more resources to be allocated to research into this problem.

DIFFERENTIAL FERTILITY AND INTELLIGENCE

Chairman: Dr Fraser Roberts

SOCIAL AND ECONOMIC DIFFERENTIALS IN FERTILITY

B. Benjamin
Statistics Division, Ministry of Health, London.

In the years since World War II demography has become a much more developed science than previously. Not only has there been accumulated a wealth of information about the determinants and consequences of population changes and about the character of these changes in populations at different stages of economic development, but demographers have become much better equipped to extract meaning from this information. As a result some early generalizations have been shown to be true not at all times but only at certain times in historical development, and, in any case, to be over-simplifications. This is especially true of the interrelationship of poverty and large families. While there undoubtedly was a time when large families helped the poor to become poorer and when the poor could command few other interests than procreation, it is no longer so in Britain ; nor does it apply to any other society in an advanced state of economic development. It need not necessarily be true of a developing country, since it is at least technically possible with modern contraceptive measures to break the vicious circle of high fertility and a low level of living. Moreover, in speaking of large families the term ' large ' has to be related to subjective parental desires rather than to more objective measures such as replacement levels. As will be shown later, we can now generalize more accurately by saying that the lowest social classes tend to have more children than their collectively expressed ideal, while the highest classes tend to come closer to their ideal family size, the ideals differing from class to class. More important still, it will be demonstrated that what happens when fertility is entirely under voluntary control is very different from what happens before this condition is reached. In speaking of fertility differentials in a society, it will therefore be necessary to specify the general extent of voluntary fertility control obtaining in that society.

It will also be necessary to distinguish between economic differentials in fertility at a point of time when 'ideal' family sizes can be regarded as stable for particular social strata, and changes in fertility as associated with economic changes such as trade cycles or sharp rises in unemployment, when 'ideals' may change differently for different social strata.

One important assumption can be made. Since there is no evidence of any real differences in natural fecundity between social groups, it can be assumed that differences in actual fertility must arise from amount of exposure to childbearing, i.e. age at marriage, mortality during the childbearing age, frequency of coitus, and, especially, the degree of practice of contraception.

In Great Britain the first detailed fertility inquiry derived from the 1911 Census (adequate information from vital registration could not be obtained until the passage of the 1938 Population (Statistics) Act). At this census the Registrar General introduced the concept of social classes (eight broad occupational groups). The 1911 Census analysis demonstrated a marked social class gradient in family size (children born). For marriages of completed fertility (wives aged forty-five or over at census) the average family size rose from 3·7 in Class I (the 'upper and middle class') to 5·0 for Class III (skilled workmen) and 5·3 for Class V (unskilled workers). A figure of 6·3 was shown for miners. These differences were not greatly affected when account was taken of differences in the age and marriage duration structure of the groups. The census inquiry also showed that the differences between the social classes increased during the latter half of the nineteenth century. It is assumed that this reflected the fact that the knowledge of contraceptive methods became accessible to the better educated and better circumstanced section of society first. It was suspected, and later became clear, that a decline in fertility was then occurring in all classes, particularly in the high fertility classes. We now know that, as a result of legislation against child labour, the latter were finding large families more of an economic burden and, as a result of declining infant mortality, less necessary for the achievement of a desired number of survivors. The gap between the classes was already beginning to narrow.*

When the Royal Commission on Population was set up in 1944 there had been no intervening fertility census since 1911 and the comprehensive vital statistics, collected under the Population (Statistics) Act, dated only from 1938. The Royal Commission therefore set up an organization to carry out a family census, on a voluntary basis, in a 10 per cent sample of married women. In order to examine social and economic differences, women were divided into nine categories according to husband's occupation. For women first married in 1900–09 the number of children born averaged 2·33 for (the wives of) professional workers, 2·64 for employers, 2·37 for salaried workers, 2·89 for non-manual wage earners, 3·96 for manual wage earners and 4·45 for labourers, against an overall average of 3·53. Thus the largest family size was 26 per cent above and the lowest 34 per cent below the overall mean.

For marriages of 1920–24 (a marriage cohort later by 15–20 years) the overall average family size had fallen to 2·42, the spread now extending from salaried employees at 1·65, through professional workers at 1·75 (no longer the smallest), to 1·97 for non-manual wage earners and 3·5 for labourers. Taken at its face value this is a relatively wider spread, but, if one has regard to the two dominant groups of non-manual and manual wage earners, the range for both marriage cohorts remains the same, viz. from 20 per cent below the all categories mean for non-manual to 12 per cent above for manual wage earners.

* In all these calculations childlessness in married couples is taken into account (i.e. family size *zero* is included in the average), but not differences in the proportion of women in different social groups who marry (and who appear in the denominator of the average). This proportion is lower in the lowest social class than in the highest but not, in the classes used here, substantially so—certainly not to such an extent as to counter-balance, in terms of reproduction of the group, the much larger differential in family size. We have been observing (1951) a family size in the highest social class which is two-thirds that of the lowest, at a time when, at most, the marriage proportion is only of the order of 10 per cent higher. Differential marriage incidence is not an important factor in this particular context. (A short note on this point appeared in *The Eugenics Review* 1966. **58**, 49–50.)

Because of the shorter durations of more recent marriages it was not possible for the Family Census Report to carry this analysis further in terms of completed fertility, but the statistics for ten-year and shorter durations of marriage suggested that the fall in fertility between World Wars I and II had been slightly more marked for the manual group. The gap had narrowed.

The fertility report of the 1951 Census, unfortunately the most recent available, started from this position, viz. that the fertility differences between social groups increased during the second half of the nineteenth century, were stabilized for several decades and then narrowed for couples married in the 1930s. The census made it possible to bring into the analysis some new dimensions, notably education (or more exactly, the age of cessation of full-time education) and urbanization, as well as, as in previous analyses, age at marriage. The last two factors had little to contribute to the persisting pattern of family size increasing from Social Class I (professional and managerial) to Social Class V (unskilled workers), though again the gradient was less steep (85 to 125 per cent of overall average) for women of census age under fifty than for women of census age 45–49 with completed fertility (75 to 132 per cent of overall average). The gap was still tending to narrow.

For the more recent fertility experience Social Class I (professional) appeared relatively more fertile, with current fertility equal to the mean for all groups combined. The Report emphasized the significance of the fact that family size in this class, probably the class which started the historic decline in fertility, had apparently begun to rise in relation to the general average, though the available facts, based on a single year preceding the census, were then inconclusive and needed to be confirmed. The trend has not yet been confirmed because the 1961 Census results are not yet available.

When one looked at the picture in greater detail it appeared that the groups with the largest mean family size and smallest proportion of infertility were the manual workers, especially the unskilled and semiskilled, members of the armed forces (other ranks), and farmers and agricultural workers. At the other end of the scale were clerical workers, managerial and professional workers, traders and shop assistants.

An important new fact, though not an unexpected one, brought out by the 1951 Census, was that fertility varied inversely with terminal education age, and this variation was slightly more consistent than variation of fertility with socio-economic group. When standardized for marriage age and socio-economic group, the index of family size decreased from 101 per cent of the overall mean for those leaving full-time education at ages under 15 to 89 per cent for those pursuing full-time education to ages 20 and over. There were some exceptions, however. For example, for the higher professional administrative and managerial occupations the mean family size of those whose full-time education lasted until after their twentieth birthday was in fact the greatest.

As regards industrial variation the highest fertility was that of wives whose husbands were in the mining and quarrying group, and was associated with their tendency to marry young. Other high fertility groups were those engaged in building and contracting, metal manufacture, and agriculture and forestry.

Married women who were themselves gainfully occupied had lower fertility than those who were not, but of course it is impossible to say which was the cause and which the effect.

There we must leave Great Britain and, for more recent Western experience, turn to the United States of America, where in the last few years there have been many intensive surveys of the growth of families. The USA has shared the experience of some other Western countries, Britain in particular, of an upward fluctuation in numbers of births. In the USA, as here, this has been mainly the result of a trend towards earlier marriage and narrower birth spacing (family-building in shorter time) and, until the marriage cohorts involved have reached longer durations of marriage, it will not be known whether this represents a real increase in fertility as distinct from an alteration in timing. The general impression is that if there is any increase in fertility it is not a trend to larger families but a decrease in childlessness and an increase in families of two, three, and four children. A. A. Campbell (reporting to the World Population Conference 1965 on

'Recent fertility trends in the USA and Canada') has preferred to use educational attainment as an indication of socio-economic level, because this seldom changes after childbearing has started. He has found that the upward trend in fertility has been strongest in college graduates as compared with those not proceeding beyond high school and has narrowed the gap that previously existed between the two groups. Comparing marriage cohorts of 1901–05 and those of 1926–30, the ratio of family size for college graduates as compared with those who failed to complete elementary school has fallen from 2·4 to 1·4. There has been a change in attitude. Few couples want a childless marriage and the majority at all educational levels want to have two to four children. The change is especially marked in the better educated. This change too has occurred at a time when surveys have shown that 96 per cent of couples with normal reproductive capacity have used or intend to use some method to limit fertility, i.e. when fertility is generally under voluntary control.

Campbell remarks that this last condition means that fertility should be more sensitive to social and economic influences, and he quotes Dudley Kirk [2] as showing that more couples marry and more try to have children when economic conditions are good. Marriages and births are often postponed when conditions are less favourable. This mainly effects timing rather than the total number of children.

With regard to the question of voluntary fertility control, Westoff [3] reports that "while most pregnancies in the USA are unplanned, most couples seem to have the number of children they want", because the effectiveness with which contraception is practised and the proportion practising contraception both increase dramatically as desired family size is approached and achieved. In the USA all socio-economic groups (and religious groups) are in favour of some control, but family planning attitudes which were previously differentiated by social factors are now converging. Large differences no longer exist in income or occupational groups as such or between urban and rural groups; the main differentiating factors are now education and religion. The less well educated, however, no longer lack information or interest in contraceptive methods. It is true that problems of excess fertility are still severe at the most deprived social levels, but this is the only exception to the general narrowing of social and economic differentials in fertility. With regard to educational differentials, Westoff states that although women of different educational accomplishments are similar in the number of children they desire, they are quite different in the number of children they have had and in the total number they actually expect.

In Japan, another country of advanced economic development, the same trends are found by Kimura.[1] Rapid economic development there has resulted in a decline in the fertility of groups which have hitherto experienced high fertility. This trend to lower fertility has been accompanied by a narrowing of social differentials; in particular there has been little decline in the fertility of the professional and managerial group, which was already low. In 1955 the standard deviation of family size according to occupation of father was 0·90 (average family size 3·0); in 1960 this had contracted to 0·16 (average family size 2·3). Opinion surveys on fertility show a continuing decline in the rates of childbearing and a convergence among the various social and economic strata, the dominant ‘ motives ’ being a desire for higher educational attainment for children, a desire for a higher level of living, and a desire to protect maternal health, in that order of priority.

Generally, then, it appears that, while social and economic fertility differentials persist in developed economies, their intensity is very much reduced as soon as a state is reached when fertility is entirely under voluntary control and when there is much more correspondence between idealized family size, which maximizes educational and social opportunity for the children, and the actual family size achieved. Transient economic changes themselves affect the timing of marriages and births but apparently do not affect long-term desires or their eventual achievement. We can now speak of fertility much more in terms of people's desires and motives. Whether the educational bias in this motivation means that the social differences in fertility, which are now narrowing, may actually be reversed we do not yet know.

REFERENCES

1. KIMURA, M. 1966. Current fertility patterns in Japan. In *World Population Conference 1965*. United Nations. In press.
2. KIRK, DUDLEY. 1960. *Influence of Business Cycles on Marriage and Birth Rates in Demographic and Economic Changes in Developed Countries*. Princeton University Press, pp. 241–260.
3. WESTOFF, C. F. 1966. Fertility control in the United States. In *World Population Conference 1965*. United Nations. In press.

DIFFERENTIAL FERTILITY BY INTELLIGENCE

C. O. CARTER
Clinical Genetics Research Unit, Institute of Child Health, London

THE biologist sees the development of a child's observed operational intelligence as due to the interaction of its genetic endowment and its environment—environment being first intra-uterine, and later—after birth—including home, neighbourhood, education and other social factors. The biologist knows that the genetic endowment of an individual child cannot now, and perhaps never will, be precisely measurable independent of the environment, and that, even if it were possible to measure a child's genetic endowment for intelligence at say age ten, this would probably provide little information about the genes controlling intellectual development between the ages of ten and twenty years. He is, however, prepared to attempt to assess in a particular group of children at say age ten, or of young adults, at say age twenty, what proportion of the total variance in the scores they make in a particular intelligence test is due to additive genetic variance. Mr Huntley will be discussing some of the methods available in the next paper of this Symposium. The general concept is that the total variance in the particular population, that is the sum of the squares of the deviations of individual scores from the population mean, is made up of the variance due to genetic variation plus the variance due to differing environmental experience plus the variance due to genetic-environmental interaction. This may be represented as:

$$V_p = V_g + V_e + V_i.$$

The interaction term V_i is included to allow for the fact, well known in biology, that a particular difference in environment may have different effects on different genotypes and vice versa. Professor Thoday [15] gave some examples at our Symposium in 1964.

In assessing the significance of a differential fertility, either positive or negative, by social class or other criteria, the biologist will probably be most concerned about its implications for the genetic component in intelligence, that is the contribution of the differential to the mean level and the variance of this genetic component in future generations. If the differential by social class has no significance in terms of the genetic component for intelligence, those concerned with educational standards may well welcome a positive differential fertility by social class, whereby an increasing proportion of children in each generation are born into homes in which they will be encouraged to educate themselves to their full academic potential. But if there is differential fertility in terms of the genetic component for intelligence this could compensate for a fall in environmental standards, and —what is more relevant— could greatly potentiate the effect of a rise in environmental standards. Many gifted men and women have shown that the lack of any secondary education, and the lack of a cultured home background, is no absolute bar to great artistic, scientific and managerial achievement.

Before going further it will be helpful to illustrate, in admittedly over-simplified form, the geneticists' concept of the kind of mechanism that underlies the genetic variance in the population for intellectual development. It is very probable that the genetic component in the development of operational intelligence is polygenic, that it depends on many pairs of gene loci on many different chromosome pairs, and that there are multiple alleles, i.e. alternative forms of a gene, at most of these gene loci. A very simple model for the situation at one of these gene loci is that in which there are three alleles— the commonest with say a frequency of one half, which tends to give average intelligence, say an IQ score of 100 ; another with frequency of one quarter which tends to give a score 10 points above average intelligence ; the third also with frequency one quarter which tends to give a score 10 points below average intelligence. If marriage is not assortative for intelligence, this would give a population distribution of intelligence as in Figure 1, one-sixteenth of the population being very bright or very dull, with scores of 120 and 80 respectively, one quarter being moderately bright or moderately dull, scoring 110 and 90 respectively, and half being at or about the average score of 100.

Bringing more gene loci with similar effects into the model spreads the variance and smooths the distribution. Figure 2 shows the distribution given by two gene loci.

Environmental differences would further increase the variance and further smooth the distribution. The distribution of the random six-day sample of about 1000 in the 1947 Scottish survey [11] is shown in Figure 3.

What we are interested in to-day is the relation between one generation and the next. If marriage is not assortative for intelligence, i.e. there is no tendency for like-intelligences to marry each other, and if there is no differential fertility, on the one gene locus model the relationship between fathers

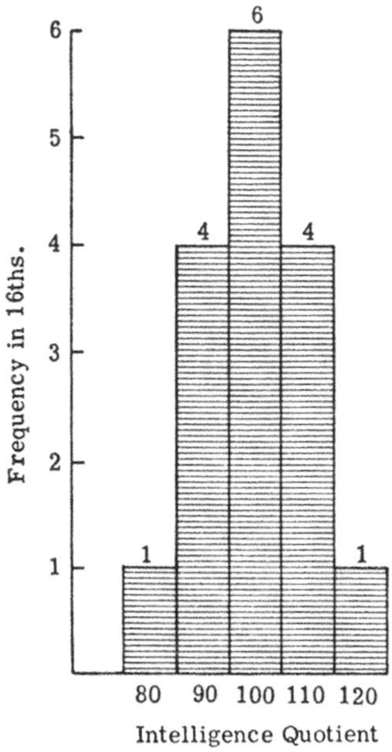

FIGURE 1

THE DISTRIBUTION OF INTELLIGENCE PRODUCED BY 3 ALLELES AT A SINGLE GENE LOCUS and sons is as shown in Figure 4. These could just as well have been mothers and sons, or fathers and daughters, or mothers and daughters.

The mean intelligence of the sons of the bright fathers and of the dull fathers regresses halfway back to the mean of the population ; for example, the mean score of the sons of the fathers of 120 is 110, but the distribution of intelligence test score in the sons is the same as that in the fathers. To use a recent dictum of Medawar's " the population breeds true, but the individual does not . . ." If there is no differential fertility there is no change in the gene frequency between generations, and so the population distribution does not alter.

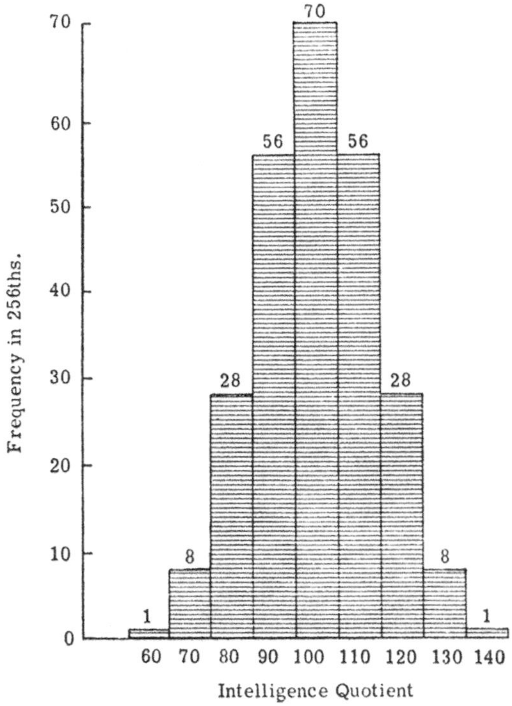

FIGURE 2

THE DISTRIBUTION OF INTELLIGENCE PRODUCED BY 3 ALLELES AT EACH OF TWO GENE LOCI

It is worth noting that on this model, only a quarter of the very bright sons are born to very bright fathers, a half—the largest proportion—come from the moderately bright fathers, and a quarter come from fathers who are only average. The average fathers contribute as many very bright sons as the very bright fathers, but the proportion of all their sons who are very bright is only one-sixteenth, whereas a quarter of the sons of the very bright fathers are also very bright. There are good genetic reasons for the old observation that the sons of very bright fathers are seldom as bright as their fathers, and conversely that the fathers of very bright sons are seldom as bright as their sons. On this model, below-average fathers have no very bright sons, though, of course, both in fact and on more complex models involving many gene loci and environmental effects such fathers would have very bright sons, but only in low proportion.

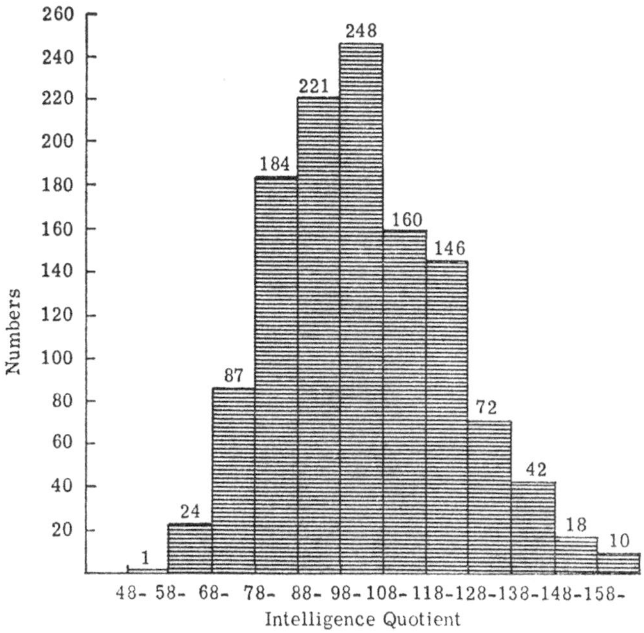

FIGURE 3

INTELLIGENCE

If there is differential fertility for the genetic element in intelligence, then there will be changes in gene frequency between generations, and both the population mean and the variance may alter. On the one gene-locus model, if of the

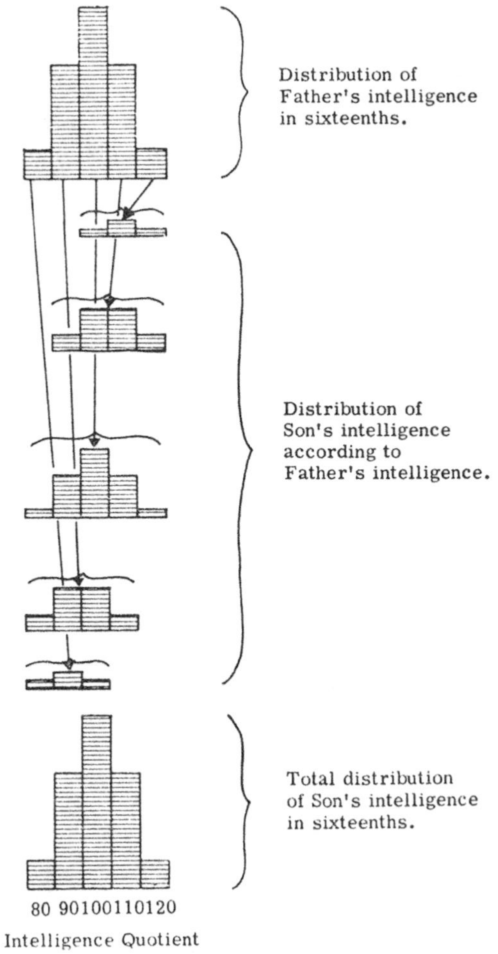

FIGURE 4

THE CONSTANCY OF THE DISTRIBUTION OF INTELLIGENCE FROM ONE GENERATION TO ANOTHER DESPITE FILIAL REGRESSION very dull fathers one-sixteenth (6·25 per cent) of the whole, had no children, and the others had an equal and compensatory increase in fertility so that the total number of sons remains unchanged, there would be 20 per cent fewer very dull sons than there were very dull fathers ; there would also be a reduction of 6·66 per cent in the number of moderately dull sons, a small—2 per cent—rise in average sons and a rise of 6·66 per cent in the number of both moderately bright sons and very bright sons. On a model in which many gene loci of additive effect are involved the effects would be much the same, though more continuous. If the very bright fathers had no children, there would be similar changes in the opposite direction. Since husband and wife almost certainly do tend to resemble each other in their genetic factors for intelligence, these changes would be intensified. If neither the very bright nor the very dull had children, then there would be no change in average intelligence between fathers and sons, but, at any rate on this simple model, the variance of the genetic-component intelligence would be rather less in the sons than in the fathers. In our 1964 Symposium Professor Mather[6] described such directional and such mobilizing selection and Dr Falconer will later be describing the kind of factors that would determine the quantitative effects of a consistent differential fertility for intelligence.

Consider now the information available as to whether there is at present any differential fertility for intelligence. First there is the indirect evidence from the massive Census data for differential fertility by father's occupation, which Dr Benjamin has been discussing. He has shown that, while there has been differential fertility by father's occupation, the picture is changing and there are indications that when all families are planned we may have a positive differential fertility by social class. The differential might already have changed further than the Census data suggest, as these are based on wives and give no information on the men in each occupation who do not marry. What significance has this for the genetic component for intelligence ? Certainly there is a strong correlation between a man's occupation and his intelligence test score, and there is also a correlation, less marked—as one would expect—because of regression, between a child's score and the occupation of his father. On a test with the mean score 100 and standard deviation 15, one finds that the scores of children of fathers in Social Class I average about 120, the children of fathers in Social Class II about 112, the children of fathers in Social Class III about 100, the children of fathers in Social Class IV about 99, and the children of fathers in Social Class V about 93. These are big differences and in part they are environmentally caused; but in part too they are genetic. Perhaps the best evidence for environmental causation of such differences comes from studies of children adopted early in infancy,[5] and where there has been no deliberate matching of natural and adopting mother. Differences are found in intelligence test score of the adopted children by social class of adopting father, and these may be attributed to environment; but the variance of intelligence of these adopted children by social class of adopting father is much less than that among own children, where both genetic and environmental differences contribute to the variance. Studies of twins, particularly monozygotic twins reared apart,[81,4] also provide good evidence that the different means and distributions of intelligence test score by occupation of father depend both on environmental and on genetic differences. Monozygotic twins reared apart from infancy show differences of intelligence test score in the direction to be expected from the environmental standards of the homes, but these differences are considerably less than those seen among parents' own children.

Scientific evidence apart, it is, I think, inevitable in our social system that some of the differences in intelligence test score by social class should be due to genetic variation. Sociologists who doubt this show more ingenuity than judgement. Within a family of brothers and sisters, with polygenic inheritance there should be much variation in the genetic component for intellectual development. (With no tendency for like to marry like for intelligence, the genetic variance within families should be as much as half the total population genetic variance.) Very considerable variation in observed intelligence within families is seen in practice, and the children who are much above the family average will tend to move up the socio-economic scale, and those much below to move down, though characteristics other than intelligence will play a part in this. Dr Gibson [16] reported at our Symposium in 1964 some direct evidence for this process in his pilot survey from Cambridge. It is probable, then, that a positive differential fertility by social class is to be welcomed on genetic as well as purely educational grounds.

But such a differential fertility is not necessarily a fact, and it would be more informative if we had good data relating fertility directly to intelligence. There are very good data relating a child's intelligence test score to the number of his (or her) brothers and sisters.[11, 12] These consistently show quite a strong negative correlation (between −0·2 and −0·3), and the negative correlation held even with social classes, except perhaps in Social Class I. It was these findings that led before the last war to the fear of a decline in national intelligence. There is in fact no direct evidence of such a decline ; the two Scottish surveys of eleven-year-olds in 1932 and 1947 showed that there had been a small improvement in mean intelligence level of eleven-year-olds in Scotland,[13] though this small gain, in my opinion, was probably not at all genetic, since environmental gains over these fifteen years were known to have led to increases in height, weight and physical maturity at that age. One reason why the negative correlation might be misleading was suggested by Haldane in 1949,[11] reviewing for publication his evidence to the Royal Commission on Population. He noticed that while one can reasonably draw inferences from children's intelligence and the number of their sibs as to the relationship of fertility and intelligence for those individuals in the parental generation who have had children, they tell one nothing about the members of the parental generation who have had no children at all. In fact there is now evidence that the marriage rate and the proportion of married with no children is relatively low for the very dull. Another reason why caution must be exercised in drawing genetic inferences from the relationship of a child's IQ and the number of his sibs is that very probably membership of a large family depresses a child's intelligence test score for environmental reasons, particularly on the more verbal tests.[9] What is needed, therefore, is a number of studies which directly relate an individual's intelligence test score, preferably estimated about the age of sixteen, to his or her subsequent reproductive performance. Some studies of this kind from America, a generation ago, are interesting because in contrast to the studies within sibships they show little correlation either way between an individual's IQ and his or her fertility ; but these studies were on a small scale and among selected groups.

TABLE I

AVERAGE NUMBER OF OFFSPRING OF 29-YEAR-OLD SWEDES BY INTELLIGENCE TEST SCORE

	SCORE	NUMBER	PER CENT MARRIED	MEAN NUMBER OF OFFSPRING
	Secondary	356	66·0	0·63
Primary	$\geqslant$ 100	470	71·9	0·69
Primary	50–99	2077	68·0	0·75
Primary	0–49	1135	57·1	0·66
	TOTAL SAMPLE	4038	65·2	0·711

More recently Quensel in Sweden[10] used the census of 1953 to measure the reproductive performance at age twenty-nine years of a little over 2000 national service recruits from Southern Sweden aged twenty-four when called up in 1944. Their intelligence was measured at recruitment on a test on which the average score is about 70. The recruits were placed in four groups, a dull group scoring 0–49, an average group scoring 50–99, a bright group scoring 100 or more, with only primary education, and another bright group who had had secondary education. The fertility findings are shown in Table I.

The greatest number of children per 100 mean at age twenty-nine were born to the average group, and these also had the biggest average family size; the dull group had fewer children than either the average group or the bright group and this is essentially due to their low *marriage* rate; the average family size of the dull individuals who married was relatively high. The bright group have the highest proportion married and the highest proportion with at least one child; their mean family size is smaller than that of the group of average intelligence, but they married a bit later and appear to be catching them up. The fourth group, those with selective secondary education, many of whom were training for the professions, at present have relatively small families; they understandably marry later and start their families later, but it is known from other studies of Swedish matriculants [7] that their proportion ultimately married and their fertility is higher than the population average. Professor Quensel hopes to follow this group further when their families are more complete, but this study already shows clearly the importance of marriage rate.

Two more recent studies from America deal with completed or nearly completed families. Higgins, Reed and Reed [2] three years ago, from a mass of family data which started with mentally retarded index patients, analysed the fertility of those for whom school intelligence test scores could be discovered. They too showed that marriage rate was an important statistic in estimating fertility by intelligence. Excluding the immediate family of the index patients and including only the individuals who had married, they found overall a negative correlation of intelligence and family size. The very bright and the moderately bright individuals had larger families than the average, but the dull and very dull had an even greater excess of children. However, if one included the unmarried members of the family, this negative correlation disappeared and there was a positive relationship of intelligence and family size. The relationship is shown in Table II. Fertility is highest among the very bright, but there is a second peak among the dull.

There are inevitably some uncertainties about the study; there is the question, for example, of the randomness of the sample for whom intelligence test scores were available, and so, though the conclusions are probably correct, it is satisfactory to have some more direct confirmation from the last study which I wish to quote.

Two years ago, Bajema [1] reported from Kalamazoo County

in Michigan, USA, a study in which he traced alive or dead over 85 per cent of the 1100-odd white native-born men and women born between 1916 and 1917, who had attended the sixth grade of the Public School system, where they all had an intelligence test at average age of 11½ years ; the average score was 102. The 14 per cent untraced did not differ significantly in sex ratio or intelligence from those traced. The subjects themselves showed the usual negative correlation, about −0·26, between test score and size of their sibship. But

TABLE II

AVERAGE NUMBER OF OFFSPRING PER INDIVIDUAL IN RELATION TO IQ MINNESOTA (Higgins, Reed and Reed, 1962.)

IQ RANGE	NUMBER	MEAN NO. OF OFFSPRING
>130	25	2·96
116–130	269	2·45
101–115	778	2·26
86–100	583	2·16
71–85	208	2·39
56–70	74	2·46
0–55	29	1·38
TOTAL SAMPLE	1966	2·27

between the subject's test score and their reproductive performance there was a small *positive* correlation and again a striking bimodal relationship, with highest fertility among the very bright and the moderately dull and lowest fertility (apart from the few very dull) among the average group. His findings are summarized in Table III.

In the survey of Reed and his colleagues,[2] which was not restricted by colour or birthplace, it was the low marriage rate of the very dull that was responsible for their low fertility. In Bajema's series the low average family size of the very dull was partly due to a low marriage rate, but rather more to a relatively high proportion of married but childless ; but the overall picture is essentially similar to that of Reed and his colleagues.

It would be most helpful to have similar data on a large scale for Britain. The Scottish 1947 six-day sample would be most suitable for a study of this kind. But on the basis of the more recent social class data for this country and the relatively high fertility in recent years of selected group of high intelligence, such as women with first class honours degrees from British Universities [3] or Scholars of Winchester,[4] it is probable that the relationship between fertility and intelligence is now similar to that shown in Reed and Bajema's studies from America and has the form of the continuous line shown in Figure 5.

TABLE III

AVERAGE NUMBER OF OFFSPRING PER INDIVIDUAL IN RELATION TO IQ—TERMAN GROUP TEST

KALAMAZOO COUNTY, MICHIGAN (C. Bejama, 1963)

IQ RANGE	NUMBER	MEAN NO. OF OFFSPRING
⩾ 130	23	3·00
120–129	59	2·44
105–119	282	2·24
95–104	318	2·02
80–94	267	2·46
69–79	30	1·50
TOTAL SAMPLE	979	2·24

I think it probable that for deliberately planned children (planned in the sense of total number planned even if spacing is not always planned) there is in fact a uniformly direct relationship between observed intelligence and fertility, and that the second peak at IQ below 95 is due to this dull group still having a substantial proportion of unplanned and often unwanted children.

The projected planned fertility for a series such as Bajema's is shown in the broken line in Figure 5, and assumes the fertilities shown in Table III to change to 2·9, 2·4, 2·0, 1·8, 1·6 and 1·0 in descending order of intelligence. We may reasonably expect these unplanned children to become progressively fewer, provided that the dull and the very dull group are given all necessary help to plan their families. This will give a continuous positive correlation between intelligence and fertility.

Such a relationship is likely to lead to a rise in the average levels of observed intelligence based probably on both genetic and environmental advances. The genetic gain would be slow in sociological perspective but rapid seen on the time scale or human evolution. In my opinion, this is to be welcomed, and a wise society will not only provide all the help that it can to help its duller members to plan the size of their families,

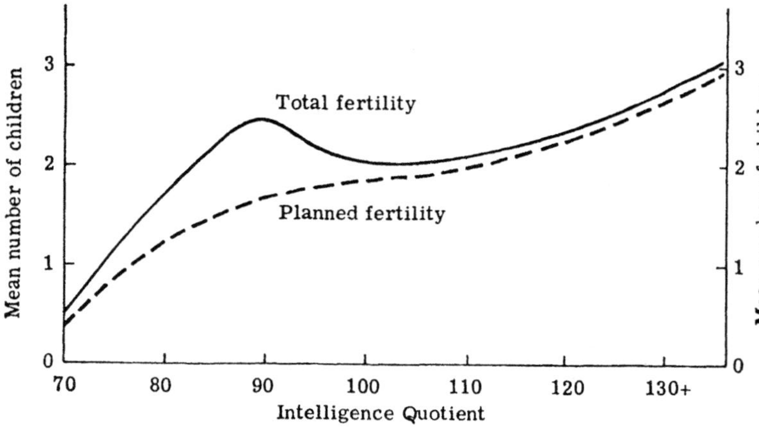

FIGURE 5

SUGGESTED PRESENT RELATIONSHIP OF PLANNED AND EXCESS FERTILITY IN BRITAIN

but will also encourage its most gifted to plan a family size above replacement rate.

DISCUSSION

DR CARTER said, in reply to questioners, that there was direct evidence for the gap between the actual and the desired size of family by social class. Social Class I's family size was far nearer to their ideal than that of Social Class IV. By IQ there was little direct evidence. In a study in Aberdeen, mothers who were having their first babies were asked how many they would like to have: though the sample was a small one, it was of interest that the more intelligent women wanted larger families irrespective of the occupations of their husbands.

In the Minnesota Survey, the data were for one parent; there was a correlation of about 0·5 between the IQ of husband and wife, and this would increase the effect of any differential fertility by intelligence.

It was difficult to say to what extent an increase in average intelligence from one generation to another could be attributed to genetic changes; it was of the order of one to two points per generation, so that if there had been a ten-point rise only a small part of this could be due to a genetic change.

REFERENCES

1. Bajema, C. J. 1963. Estimation of the direction and intensity of natural selection in relation to human intelligence by means of the intrinsic rate of natural increase. *Eugen. Quart.* **10**, 175.
2. Higgins, J., Reed, E. and Reed, S. 1962. Intelligence and family size: a paradox resolved. *Eugen. Quart.* **9**, 84.
3. Hubback, J. 1955. The fertility of graduate women. *Eugen. Rev.* **47**, 2.
4. Hutton, K. 1953. Intelligence quotients and differential fertility: some observations from Winchester College. *Eugen. Rev.* **44**, 205.
5. Leahy, A. M. 1935. Nature, nurture and intelligence. *Genet. Psychol. Monogr.* **17**, 236.
6. Mather, K. 1965. Medicine and natural selection in man. In *Biological Aspects of Social Problems.* (Ed. J. E. Meade and A. S. Parkes.) Edinburgh. Oliver and Boyd.
7. Moberg, S. 1950. Marital status and family size among matriculated persons in Sweden. *Popul. Stud.* **4**, 115.
8. Newman, H. H., Freeman, F. N. and Holzinger, K. J. 1937. *Twins: A Study of Heredity and Environment.* Chicago. University of Chicago Press.
9. Nisbet, J. D. 1953. *Family Environment: A Direct Effect of Family Size on Intelligence.* Occasional Papers on Eugenics, No. 8. London. Cassell.
10. Quensel, C. T. E. 1957. The interrelationship of marital status, fertility, family size and intelligence test scores. *Popul. Stud.* **11**, 234.
11. Royal Commission on Population. 1950. *Papers.* Vol. V. London. H.M.S.O.
12. Scottish Council for Research in Education. 1953. *Social Implications of the 1947 Scottish Mental Survey.* London. University of London Press.

13. SCOTTISH COUNCIL FOR RESEARCH IN EDUCATION. 1949. *The Trend of Scottish Intelligence.* London. University of London Press.
14. SHIELDS, J. 1962. *Monozygotic Twins Brought up Apart and Brought up Together.* London. Oxford University Press.
15. THODAY, J. M. 1965. Geneticism and environmentalism. In *Biological Aspects of Social Problems.* (Ed. J. E. Meade and A. S. Parkes.) Edinburgh. Oliver and Boyd.
16. YOUNG, M. and GIBSON, J. B. 1965. Social mobility and fertility. In *Biological Aspects of Social Problems.* (Ed. J. E. Meade and A. S. Parkes.) Edinburgh. Oliver and Boyd.

HERITABILITY OF INTELLIGENCE

R. M. C. Huntley

Clinical Genetics Research Unit, Institute of Child Health, London

The concept of heritability is not difficult to define. The difficulties appear when one attempts to estimate it for a particular characteristic in a population of human beings.

At the beginning of his paper Dr Carter spoke of operational intelligence as due to the interaction of genetic endowment and environment, this latter including all kinds of non-genetic influence—intra-uterine life, the home, education and other social factors. The genetic endowment cannot be measured independently of the environment, but it is possible to assess what proportion of the total variance of the scores on a particular intelligence test is due to additive genetic variance. This genetic proportion of the total variance is the heritability which I am attempting to assess. The ' particular ' nature of it should again be emphasized, lest the title of this paper should lead to too high expectations of the result. We cannot measure *the* heritability of intelligence once and for all. All that can be offered is an estimate of the heritability of intelligence as measured from scores obtained on a particular test by a particular group of people living at a particular time in a particular area. If any one of these were different the heritability might be different too.

Like most human characteristics, intelligence varies continuously in the population. This fact of continuous variation is an indication of a particular mode of inheritance, known as multifactorial or polygenic, meaning that the character is determined by a number of gene pairs, individually of small effect, but added together giving the final expression of the character in the individual. The same kind of variation could also be produced by the additive effect of many small environmental causes. In practice the total variability will be produced by a combination of both genetic and environmental causes of variability, each contributing a certain proportion of the total. The proportion which the additive genetic variance bears to the total variance is the heritability of the particular character in a population. We specify *additive* variance because that is the part of the genetic variance which contributes to a resemblance between parent and child, whereas non-additive variance or variance due to dominance does not. My task is to show how different estimates of heritability can be made, for intelligence, from scores made on a particular test by a particular group of people.

The approach will be to work from the fact that, in general, relatives resemble one another more than they resemble other people to whom they are not related. We shall then consider the reasons for the observed resemblances between different relatives by comparing them with resemblances we should expect to get assuming *either* genetic *or* environmental determination. Finally we shall consider the theory underlying various methods of estimating heritability and apply the relevant ones to the observed resemblances between relatives.

First, then, the resemblances we should expect to get, given continuous variation, and polygenic inheritance, between various kinds of relative. The theory for this genetic treatment of continuous variation was given by Fisher [7] in 1918, when he showed that, provided certain assumptions are realized the resemblances between relatives depend on the number of genes they share in common. Thus the genetic resemblance between father and child is a half, because a child receives half his genes from his father, and so is genetically half like him. Similarly, siblings—ordinary brothers and sisters—also share on average half their genes in common, and so are half alike. There is a genetic correlation between them of 0·50. Dizygotic (DZ) twins, being genetically no more alike than ordinary brothers and sisters, will also show a genetic resemblance of a half. Monozygotic (MZ) twins, on the other hand, are genetically identical. They share all their genes in common, so show a genetic resemblance of 1·0.

The assumptions underlying these theoretical resemblances are (i) that genetic factors alone are responsible, and no environmental influences are having any effect, (ii) that there is no dominance and (iii) that mating is random, i.e. there is no tendency for like to marry like, resulting in a correlation between husband and wife, called *assortative mating*. In practice, of course, these assumptions are probably never all met, and complications arise in comparing observed resemblances with those based on the simple model. Dominance may or may not be involved in the inheritance of intelligence; there are certainly going to be environmental influences. Assortative mating, present in most human characteristics, is probably stronger for intelligence than for any other characteristic, certainly than for any physical one. Furthermore, these other factors will, if present, not only affect the resemblances on the simple additive gene model, but affect them in different ways. Assortative mating raises parent-child, sib-sib and DZ twin resemblances. Dominance tends to lower resemblances but does so less for sibs (and DZ twins) than it does for parent and child. Environmental influences can have both effects. In general relevant environmental differences between relatives will lower the resemblance between them expected on genetic grounds, and so lower the correlation. But this is on the assumption that, everybody, irrespective of whether they are related or not, has an equal chance on average of experiencing the various kinds of environmental conditions. Again this is an assumption which may rarely be realized in human populations. Just as a genetic resemblance between relatives arises from the fact that relatives share more genes in common than unrelated people, so, if relatives share environmental conditions in common, there will be an environmental resemblance between them which may mimic or be even higher than the expected genetic ones.

In fact, an environmental hypothesis can be set up alongside the genetic one. It is probably a reasonable hypothesis that the environments of twins, although lacking the precision of the expected genetic resemblances, are not as different as the environments of different sibs, nor are the environments of different sibs as different as the environments of parents on the one hand and their children on the other. Also, both MZ and DZ twins, to the extent that for both kinds they are two children of the same age growing up in the same family at the same time, may be assumed to be subject to much the same degree of environmental differences and similarities. So, whereas for genetic factors DZ twins and sibs share the same degree of resemblance and are less alike than MZ twins, for environmental factors the MZ and DZ twins will tend on the whole to be equally alike or equally different, and more alike than their sibs.

It is obvious, then, considering all the different influences, both genetic and non-genetic, which can affect the resemblances expected on the simple theoretical model, that any observed correlation between relatives must be interpreted with considerable caution, before using it to estimate the heritability of a character in the population. For this reason, instead of considering the correlations for intelligence in isolation, I am including resemblances obtained from the same relatives in three other characteristics, in the determination of which genetic and non-genetic factors may be thought to be playing different proportionate parts. The heritability of intelligence will then be seen in relation to the greater or lesser heritabilities of other human characteristics. These three other characters are the finger-print ridge count, height and an assessment of social maturity.

The total finger-ridge count is included because better than any other human characteristic it meets the requirements laid down by Fisher for the realization of the theoretical resemblances. The finger ridges are formed early in pregnancy and do not change thereafter. There is no need, therefore, to make any troublesome allowances for age differences between subjects. There is a small sex difference in the number of ridges but allowing for this makes no appreciable difference to the correlations. No evidence so far has shown any dominance in the inheritance of finger ridges. It is not a character which causes attraction between the sexes, so there are no complications arising from assortative mating. S. B. Holt's studies [8] have shown how closely the observed correlations in finger-ridge count fit the theoretical expectations for a character determined by polygenic inheritance alone. It is therefore a very useful measure to include with other measures on relatives, being, as Fraser Roberts [12] has suggested " a kind of sheet-anchor when the inevitable complexities that arise with other measurements are being analysed."

Height is included as a familiar example of a normal physical measurement, probably largely determined by heredity but certainly more complicated to deal with than finger-ridge counts, since it changes with age, differs between sexes, will be at least partly dependent on nutritional and climatic factors and is a character liable to an appreciable degree of assortative mating.

Intelligence as assessed here is based on a composite Vocabulary Test, using the four Vocabularies from the Terman-Merrill, the Wechsler Intelligence Scale for Children, and Raven's Mill Hill Vocabulary Forms A and B. These four scales were used together and standardized by Dunsdon and Roberts [4, 5] as one test with separate norms for boys and girls at each age from five years to fourteen years, eleven months. It is realized that there are objections to using a wholly verbal test for the assessment of intelligence and for the calculation of its heritability. However, provided it is borne in mind that it is a verbal test of intelligence, and that because of this cultural and environmental factors may influence the scores more than they would a less verbally biased test, this should not be too serious an objection.

This measurement was one of many which were taken from all the members of several hundred families for a twin family study that Dr Dunsdon and I have been doing. Since these families ranged in size from a single child to eight children, it would have been quite impracticable to administer a full-scale intelligence test in the time available. Discussing this kind of test, Dunsdon and Roberts [3] say " for the comparison of large groups vocabulary tests have manifest advantages in respect of reliability, validity, relative absence of practice effect and, above all, the amount of information obtained per unit of testing time." Such tests give " 70 per cent of the information that would be obtained using more extensive tests in 10 per cent of the testing time."

If like marries like in terms of stature, the tendency will probably be even more marked in the case of intelligence. A range of figures for assortative mating in intelligence has been reported from about 0·40 (Spuhler [14]) to more than 0·70 (see review by Alström [1]). It is probable that in western

Society the correlation for intelligence between spouses is at least as high as that between parent-child and sib-sib.

The other characteristic included for comparison with the correlations in intelligence is an assessment of social maturity using the Vineland Social Maturity Scale.[2] It assesses the individual's ability to look after his practical needs and to take responsibility in relation to his age. A social Age and Social Quotient are computed for the subject's record on the Scale.

The numbers of which the correlations for intelligence are based are 320 pairs of twins and their available non-twin siblings, making a total of 108 pairings. The numbers of sibs for height are higher because the over-fifteens are included, while for Intelligence and Social Maturity the tested age range is from five years to fourteen years, eleven months only. The numbers analysed for the finger-ridge count are smaller (103 pairs of twins). These are the three-child families only, a pair of twins and one sib. The sib has been correlated with each member of the twin pair giving 206 pairings. Of the 320 pairs of twins, 85 were Monozygotic and 235 Dizygotic; 100 DZ pairs were of unlike sex.

The twin families came from two sources. A first group was obtained with the help of the Hospital for Sick Children, Great Ormond Street. One or both twins had been a patient at the Hospital. The second group, which was needed (*a*) to increase the numbers and (*b*) as a check on whether the Hospital group was a selected one in any way, was obtained from volunteers who responded to a Television appeal for twin families living in the Greater London Area.

A correct diagnosis of zygosity is an essential part of any twin study. In this study it was carried out in two stages. An initial diagnosis was made, on the basis of marked similarity in general appearance, and essential identity in a number of physical features—hair colour, texture and form, eye colour, shape of nose, lips, ears and chin, teeth formation and types and proportion of hands and fingers—for a diagnosis of Monozygosity. If there was dissimilarity in any of these the pairs were classed as DZ. Any cases where there was real doubt (about forty pairs) were fully blood-grouped, with their parents. It was reassuring to find that in only one of these forty specially difficult cases was a wrong diagnosis demonstrated, and consequently it seems unlikely that a wrong diagnosis has been made in the remainder of the cases.

Table I shows the resemblances obtained in the four characteristics for the different relationships, together with the theoretical expected genetic resemblances. The correlations for DZ twins have been given for like-sex DZ pairs for true comparability with the inevitably like-sex MZ pairs, and then for all the DZ pairs (like plus unlike sex) for comparability with the sib pairs who are both like- and unlike-sex pairs. Husband-wife correlations are given where available. The parents of these children were measured for finger-ridge count and height, but not for intelligence or social maturity ; apart from the difficulties of testing the parents' intelligence with any accuracy, it was feared that any attempt to do so might, in a great many cases, jeopardize their whole co-operation. The figure inserted for assortative mating for intelligence is, therefore, an estimate. We do not at all know what degree of assortative mating there is for social maturity.

The correlations for the MZ twins are all very high. The ridge-count correlation of 0·96 is not significantly below the theoretical figure of 1·0, suggesting a high degree of genetic determination. Height correlation, at 0·90, is slightly lower and would be expected to be so, with non-genetic factors, perhaps slight nutritional differences, and some element of measuring error beginning to intrude. With intelligence the figure is slightly lower again, suggesting an increase in the environmental influences that are relevant in causing differences in verbal intelligence. Some part of the variability in intelligence will also be caused by measuring error in the form of unreliability of the test and of the subject measured. We know that the correlation of a child's score with his score a year later is in the region of 0·95, so the unreliability of the test score as a cause of differences between MZ twins is probably not very important. Environmental differences, then, do not appear to be affecting the intelligence scores.

In social maturity, the correlation between the MZ twins is very high. In fact at 0·97 it is suspiciously high, being,

TABLE I

RESEMBLANCES BETWEEN RELATIVES

		Observed Correlations							
Relationship	Theoretical Correlation	Number of pairs	Finger print ridge counts	Number of pairs	Height	Number of pairs	Intelligence	Number of pairs	Social maturity
MZ twins	1·0	27	0·96±0·02	85	0·90±0·02	85	0·83±0·03	85	0·97±0·01
DZ twins (like-sex)	0·5	39	0·47±0·13	135	0·57±0·06	135	0·66±0·05	135	0·89±0·02
DZ twins (all)	0·5	76	0·49±0·09	235	0·58±0·04	235	0·58±0·04	235	0·82±0·02
Sibs	0·5	206	0·51±0·05	176	0·50±0·06	108	0·58±0·06	108	0·32±0·09
Husband-wife	0·0	103	0·01±0·10	320	0·34±0·05	—	(0·50) estimated	—	Not known

if anything, higher than that for the finger-ridge count. How could a character which would seem much more likely to be subject to home, cultural and social pressures produce a resemblance between MZ twins as high as, or even higher than, that produced in a character which is highly genetically determined ? Presumably, by environmental factors which, being as similar for each member of a twin pair as their similarity in the number of genes they share in common, will produce an environmental resemblance which mimics the genetic one.

A high MZ correlation by itself, then, does not prove genetic determination. More information is needed, in order to identify the causative factor. The difficulty is partly resolved by bringing in the other DZ twin and sib correlations for comparison. On the genetic hypothesis they should be near 0·50 ; on the environmental hypothesis the DZ twins should be more like the MZ twins, while the sibs would be less alike than the twins.

The DZ twin correlations for ridge-count are 0·47 and 0·49, for like-sex, and all DZ twins respectively. By their very significant difference from the MZ correlation they fully confirm the hypothesis of wholly genetic determination. The sib-sib correlation is virtually 0·50, showing that the presumed greater difference of environment of sibs than of twins is having no effect on the resemblances in this character. For height, the DZ twin correlation is somewhat higher than 0·50 at 0·57 and 0·58, while the sib correlation is 0·50. That the sib correlation is lower than the DZ twin one is not surprising ; for, apart from possibly greater relevant environmental differences, the sibs are necessarily of different ages and at different stages of development, so that the resemblance between them may well be lower than it would be if they were all fully grown.

Assortative mating is undoubtedly helping to raise the correlations above 0·50. For height, the correlations between spouses is seen to be 0·34, whereas for finger-ridges it was not significantly different from zero. Similarly for intelligence, allowance for assortative mating will raise the expected theoretical correlations of 0·50, so that the observed correlations of 0·66, 0·58 and 0·58, for like-sexed DZ twins, all DZ twins, and sibs respectively, do not necessarily indicate non-genetic determination. However, the MZ correlation has been lowered by 0·83 by non-genetic factors, and these will also affect the DZ correlation. Therefore, either powerful influences arising from assortative mating, or marked similarity of environment of twin pairs must be tending to raise the correlations to the levels observed here.

The correlations for social maturity are of a different order from those for finger-ridges. The DZ like-sex correlation is only a little less than the MZ correlation, while when the unlike-sex twins are included there is only a small fall—to 0·82. It cannot be assortative mating which causes these very high DZ twin correlations ; for, if it were, the sib-sib correlation would also be high, whereas it is only 0·32. This character appears to support the hypothesis of wholly environmental determination nearly as strongly as the ridge-counts suggest the workings of a wholly genetic determination based on the simple theoretical model. Height, and especially intelligence, appear to fall between these two extremes.

We come now to the use of these correlations in the actual quantitative estimates of heritability—the proportion of the total population variance which is due to additive genetic variance.

Heritability estimates are distorted by the effects of assortative mating. However, assortative mating has a measurable effect on resemblances and can be allowed for. Fisher [7] showed that assortative mating raises parent-child, sib-sib and DZ twin correlations to $\frac{1}{2}(1+m)$ where m is the degree of assortative mating. The only difficulty is making allowance for assortative mating is that of knowing whether the observed husband-wife correlation is in fact *genetic* assortative mating. The mating takes place on a phenotypic level, and this does not necessarily mean that the phenotype is an accurate portrayal of the genotype. In intelligence the actual degree of assortative mating will certainly only in part be genetic, and so only a part of it will affect the correlations in the predicted manner. We are making the assumption that *half* the phenotypic resemblance between parents is genetic, and show in Table II the correlations again with this effect removed.

The ridge-count figures are unaffected. The height and intelligence figures are somewhat lower, and come much closer to those obtained for the finger-ridges. The MZ correlations are unaffected by assortative mating. MZ twins, being genetically identical anyhow, cannot be made more alike by any genetic similarity between their parents.

From the form in which the correlations appear in Table II the heritability estimates can be calculated. The methods used are two of several suggested by our next contributor,

TABLE II

RESEMBLANCES BETWEEN RELATIVES

		Correlations after allowing for effect of Genetic Assortative Mating			
Relationship	Theoretical Correlation	Finger-print ridge counts	Height	Intelligence	Social maturity
MZ twins	1·0	0·96	0·90	0·83	0·97
DZ twins (like-sex)	0·5	0·47	0·48	0·53	0·89
DZ twins (all).	0·5	0·49	0·49	0·45	0·82
Sibs	0·5	0·51	0·41	0·45	0·32

Dr Falconer,[6] in his book *Introduction to Quantitative Genetics*. He shows how the total variance can be partitioned into the variance within groups, and the variance between groups, and the two parts into their genetic and environmental components.

Thus for MZ twins all the additive genetic variance will be *between* pairs, because there are no unshared genes to cause differences within the pairs. Similarly all variance due to dominance will be between pairs, because either both twins will be affected by dominance effects, or neither will. Differences within the pairs will be environmental differences. But if these environmental differences within pairs are less than the total environmental variance in the population, there will be a portion of this total variance between the pairs—being that portion of the total variance which is common to members of the twin pairs and is an additional cause of similarity between them.

MZ and DZ twins, by virtue of being two children of the same age growing up in the same family at the same time, may be assumed, in general, to be subject to much the same degree of environmental differences and similarities. Hence in partitioning the variance for DZ twins the within-pair environmental variance component and the between-pair common environmental variance component will be the same as for MZ twins. However, DZ twins are on average genetically only half alike ; so half the additive genetic variance will be within

TABLE III

COMPOSITION OF THE COMPONENTS OF VARIANCE BETWEEN AND WITHIN PAIRS OF TWINS

	BETWEEN PAIRS	WITHIN PAIRS
MZ twins	$V_A + V_D + V_{Ec}$	V_{Ew}
DZ twins	$\frac{1}{2}V_A + \frac{1}{4}V_D + V_{Ec}$	$\frac{1}{2}V_A + \frac{3}{4}V_D + V_{Ew}$
Difference	$\frac{1}{2}V_A + \frac{3}{4}V_D$	$\frac{1}{2}V_A + \frac{3}{4}V_D$

V_A = Additive genetic variance.
V_D = Variance due to dominance.
V_{Ec} = Variance due to common environment.
V_{Ew} = Variance due to environmental differences within groups.
(from Falconer.[6] 1964, p. 184.)

pairs, and half between pairs. If there is dominance, the variance due to it will appear in both components, in unequal proportions, three-quarters of it causing differences within pairs, and one-quarter causing differences between pairs. The difference between the between-pair components for MZ and DZ twins, which is the same as the difference between the covariances of the two kinds of twins, will be equal to half the genetic variance in the population, or, if there is dominance, to half the additive variance plus three-quarters of the dominance variance.

Table III shows this partitioning of the components of variance between and within pairs of twins, and is taken, with his permission, from Dr Falconer's book.[6]

Falconer suggests therefore that the difference between the correlation coefficients of MZ and DZ twins "could be taken as an estimate of half the heritability if there were no non-additive variance . . . but since non-additive variance cannot reasonably be assumed to be absent, the difference can only be regarded as setting an upper limit to half the heritability." If there is variance due to dominance the DZ correlation will be reduced, thereby increasing the difference between the MZ and DZ correlations, and so overestimating the heritability.

Two other estimates of heritability can be made from the DZ twin and sib-sib correlations. For both kinds of relatives the covariance is made up of half the additive genetic variance plus a quarter of any dominance variance plus any variance due to common environment. The correlation coefficient will therefore estimate half the heritability if there is no variance due to common environment or dominance. If there is variance due to these factors the correlation will not give a true estimate of the heritability in the population, since the genetic resemblance is reduced by only a part of the population environmental variance, and by less than the whole of the variance due to dominance. The heritability would therefore be overestimated.

For intelligence and the three other characteristics we can, then, obtain three estimates of heritability. The first, based on the difference between MZ and DZ twin correlations, gives a true estimate, unless there is some variance due to dominance ; if there is, it will set up an upper limit to the estimate. The second, based on the DZ twin correlation, will be an upper limit according to whether it includes variance due to common environment and dominance or not. If it is greater than the first estimate, and if we assume now that there is no dominance, this will be an indication of the effect of common environment. The third estimate, based on the sib-sib correlation, will be similar to the second except in so far as the common environment of sibs is less than the common environment of DZ twins ; this will make the sib estimate lower than the twin estimate.

The heritability estimates are shown in Table IV, expressing the genetic proportion of the total variance as a percentage of that total.

All three heritability estimates for the ridge-counts are very high and consistent with each other. For this character genetic factors account for nearly all the differences in the population. Common environmental and dominance effects are not suggested by any of the estimates.

There is some variation in the estimates of height heritability, but all are high. The discrepancy between the first and second estimates could be due to the raising of the second one by common environmental variance. It is also possible that the assumption that only half the assortative mating for height was genetic was an underestimate, and that more should have been allowed for. If it were, the first estimate

TABLE IV

ESTIMATES OF HERITABILITY

Method	Characteristics: Finger-print ridge counts	Height	Intelligence	Social maturity
	Per cent	Per cent	Per cent	Per cent
$2(r_{MZ}-r_{DZ})$	98	84	60	16
$2r_{DZ}$	$\leqslant 98$	$\leqslant 98$	$\leqslant 90$	$\leqslant 164$
$2r_{SIBS}$	$\leqslant 102$	$\leqslant 82$	$\leqslant 90$	$\leqslant 64$

would be raised and the second (and third) lowered. The true heritability for height may be as much as 90 per cent. The lower heritability for sibs could be due both to their less common environment and to the fact—mentioned earlier—that being necessarily of different ages and at different stages of development they will probably resemble one another less than if they were all fully grown, or, like the twins, all of the same age.

For intelligence, there is a heritability of 60 per cent on the first estimate and a maximum of 90 per cent on each of the others. The 60 per cent is probably a true estimate and consistent with a theory that intelligence is a largely inherited characteristic, but that when, as here, the measure of it is based on a wholly verbal test, environmental factors will play a more important part than if the assessment were based on a test less dependent on an acquired knowledge and facility in the handling of words. The high and similar DZ and sib estimates also suggest a considerable degree of common environmental effect shedding its influence equally over all the members of a family, tending to make them all more alike in verbal IQ than they would be if genetic factors alone were the controlling factor in differentiating them.

The social maturity estimates are instructive as showing a character which is at the other extreme from finger-ridges in terms of genetic determination. Only 16 per cent of the total variance is due to genetic variation. The character is almost entirely the product of environmental influences, and the nonsense figure of 164 per cent for the second heritability estimate shows the very large and predominating effect of the common environment of DZ twins for this character. Two children in the same family at the same time will tend to be very much alike in degree of social maturity, irrespective of whether they are alike or unlike genetically.

At the beginning of this paper I emphasized that these heritability estimates of intelligence were based on the results obtained from a particular group of people living at a particular time in a particular part of the country and tested on a particular test, and that if any of these factors were different, the heritability might be different. This would seem to make any such particular estimate of very limited value, since it could have no general validity and comparisons with estimates from other studies obtained with different tests on different people would be rather pointless. It is surprising, however, to find how comparable the results from various studies are, though not so surprising, perhaps, in that all those I shall quote are either British or American studies, and therefore, ' western society '. Either a striking similarity is shown in the heritability estimates for intelligence, or, where there are differences, they are understandable.

Table V shows our estimates compared with four others,[9, 10, 11, 13] calculating the heritability in the same way, and making the same allowance for assortative mating. The samples come from pre-war USA and Bath, and from present-day Greater London and Scotland. The tests are either full-scale general intelligence tests combining verbal and non-verbal tests, or, in this study only, purely verbal. Estimates from twins give either 60 per cent for verbal intelligence or an expected higher figure of 76 per cent on the less verbally biased tests. The estimates from sibs are in general higher, showing, it is thought, the extra effect of common family environment. They range from our own 90 per cent or less where the verbal nature of the test is most subject to common environmental influences within families, to 82 per cent and

TABLE V

COMPARISON OF HERITABILITY ESTIMATES FOR INTELLIGENCE DERIVED FROM VARIOUS STUDIES

STUDY	Date reported	Source of material	Test(s) used	HERITABILITY (h^2) from TWINS	HERITABILITY (h^2) from SIBS
				Per cent	Per cent
Dunsdon and Huntley	1965	Greater London	Four Vocabulary	60	⩽90
Newman, Freeman and Holzinger [10]	1937	U.S.A.	Binet	76	—
Roberts [11]	1940	Bath	Advanced Otis	—	⩽82
Maxwell and Pilliner [9]	1960	Scotland	Terman-Merrill Form L	—	⩽76
Shields [13]	1962	Greater London	Vocabulary+ Dominoes	76	—

76 per cent for the Bath sibs and the Scottish sibs on general intelligence scales, less likely, probably, to be affected by common environmental influences.

It would seem, then, that certainly well over half the variability of this predominantly verbal kind of intelligence in the population is due to genetic differences between people. It is probably fair to suggest that for general operational intelligence genetic differences will be responsible for something nearer three-quarters, perhaps 70 per cent, of the total variability.

DISCUSSION

Mr Huntley emphasized that intelligence had been assessed on the basis of a comprehensive vocabulary test, and was therefore probably more likely to be influenced by cultural and environmental factors than a non-verbal test, and show a lower heritability ; which was in fact the case. With regard to the findings on the Vineland social maturity scale, the information was collected from the mothers, who on the whole were fairly intelligent people who did their best to discriminate between the twins ; in fact, it was the mothers who were aware of the differences and in most cases could not understand why other people thought the twins were alike.

REFERENCES

1. Alström, C. H. 1961. A study of inheritance of human intelligence. *Acta psychol. neurol. scand.* **36**, 175.
2. Doll, E. A. 1947. *Vineland Social Maturity Scale. Manual of Directions.* Minneapolis. Educational Test Bureau.
3. Dunsdon, M. I. and Roberts, J. A. F. 1953. The relation of the Terman-Merrill vocabulary test to mental age in a sample of English children. *Brit. J. statist. Psychol.* **6**, 61.
4. Dunsdon, M. I. and Roberts, J. A. F. 1955. A study of the performance of 2000 children on four vocabulary tests. I. Growth curves and sex differences. *Brit. J. statist. Psychol.* **8**, 3.
5. Dunsdon, M. I. and Roberts, J. A. F. 1957. A study of the performance of 2000 children on four vocabulary tests. II. Norms, with some observations on the relative variability of boys and girls. *Brit. J. statist. Psychol.* **10**, 1.
6. Falconer, D. S. 1964. *Introduction to Quantitative Genetics.* Edinburgh. Oliver and Boyd.
7. Fisher, R. A. 1918. The correlation between relatives on the supposition of Mendelian inheritance. *Trans. roy. Soc. Edin.* **52**, 399.
8. Holt, S. B. 1961. Inheritance of dermal ridge patterns. In *Recent Advances in Human Genetics* p. 101. (Ed. L. S. Penrose.) London. Churchill.
9. Maxwell, J. and Pilliner, A. E. G. 1960. The intellectual resemblance between sibs. *Ann. hum. Genet.* **24**, 23.
10. Newman, H. H., Freeman, F. N. and Holzinger, K. J. 1937. *Twins: A Study of Heredity and Environment.* Chicago. University of Chicago Press.
11. Roberts, J. A. F. 1940. Studies on a child population. V. The resemblance in intelligence between sibs. *Ann. Eugen.* **10**, 293.

12. Roberts, J. A. F. 1961. Multifactorial inheritance in relation to human traits. *Brit. med. Bull.* **17**, 241.
13. Shields, J. 1962. *Monozygotic Twins Brought up Apart and Brought up Together*. London. Oxford University Press.
14. Spuhler, J. N. 1962. Empirical studies on quantitative human genetics. In *Proceedings of the Seminar on the Use of Vital and Health Statistics for Genetic and Radiation Studies* p. 241. New York. United Nations.

GENETIC CONSEQUENCES OF SELECTION PRESSURE

D. S. FALCONER

Agricultural Research Council, Unit of Animal Genetics, Institute of Animal Genetics, Edinburgh

MY role in this Symposium is to look at the problem of differential fertility from the point of view of a quantitative geneticist. As far as the problem of intelligence is concerned I shall have to keep to a strictly theoretical level because I know little about the evidence. I shall assume that there really is a fertility differential for intelligence, and that the problem of what effect this apparent selection will have on the intelligence of future generations is a real one. The evidence reviewed by Dr Carter in his contribution to this Symposium encourages the belief that the fertility differential is positive, and not negative as it used to be supposed. What I have to say applies equally, whether the apparent selection is for increased or for decreased intelligence.

There can be no doubt that intelligence, however it may be measured, is to some degree inherited, and that most of the genetically determined variation is multifactorial, i.e. due to many genes each with small effects. The power of selection to change almost any characteristic with multifactorial inheritance within a few generations has been abundantly proved by laboratory experiments, and evidence of its efficacy over longer periods of time can readily be seen in the great variety among our breeds of domestic animals.

In view of the overpowering evidence of the efficacy of selection it may seem inevitable that human intelligence must change as a result of the selection apparently being applied to it through the differential fertility. This conclusion, however though possibly true, would not be justified by the evidence at present available. My object now is to explain why it is not a valid conclusion, and to show what additional information we need in order to predict the change of intelligence resulting from differential fertility. I shall first explain how the response to artificial selection is predicted, which is well understood and substantiated by experiment, and then introduce the modifications needed to predict the response to natural selection. It will not be possible to explain fully all the underlying genetical ideas, nor to demonstrate in full the derivation of all the mathematical expression. Details of artificial selection will be found in Lerner [7] and Falconer,[2] and more sophisticated accounts of the selection process, including natural selection, are given by Crow and Kimura [1] and Kempthorne.[5]

ARTIFICIAL SELECTION

The prediction that can be made is of the change in the mean value of the criterion of selection between one generation and the next. The criterion of selection in a laboratory experiment is usually a measurement, such as weight or test-score, which is the ' character ' selected. All individuals of a generation are measured and the best are chosen, on the basis of this measurement, to be parents of the next generation.

For the prediction of the response only two parameters are required—the heritability of the character selected, and the selection differential applied. The heritability, symbolized as h^2, expresses the degree to which the character is inherited, and is defined as the additive genetic variance, V_G, as a proportion of the total phenotypic variance, V_P, i.e. $h^2 = V_G/V_P$. (The symbol G will be used throughout as a subscript to denote genetic variance and correlation, though in every case it refers to the additive, and not to the total, genetic component.) The heritability is estimated from the degree of resemblance between relatives.

The selection differential, S, is the mean superiority of the individuals selected, over the mean of the generation to which they belong, and is a measure of the intensity of the selection applied. If the parents differ in their contribution of offspring to the next generation, as they commonly do through differences of fertility, allowance must be made for this in calculating the selection differential. The superiority of each selected individual is weighted by its relative contribution to the next generation, and the selection differential is the weighted mean superiority. Thus

$$S = \frac{1}{N} \Sigma \left[\frac{f}{\bar{f}} (X - \bar{X}) \right] \tag{1}$$

where X is the value of the character in a selected individual, f is the number of offspring it contributes to the next generation, $\bar{f}$ and $\bar{X}$ the means of f and X in the population, and N is the number of selected individuals.

The response, R, or the change in the character selected brought about by one generation of selection, is then equal to the product of the heritability and the selection differential:

$$R = h^2 S \tag{2}$$

In principle this prediction is valid for only one generation because the selection itself alters the genetic properties—specifically the heritability—of the population. In practice, however, the heritability changes only slowly and the prediction is reliable for up to five or ten generations, or even longer.

An example of the predicted and observed responses to artificial selection is illustrated in Figure 1. This shows the results of selection in mice for increased susceptibility to the induction of lung tumours by urethane, the criterion of selection being the number of tumours induced by a standard dose. Over the whole experiment the prediction was very accurate, though for any single generation it was less reliable on account of sampling variation and unavoidable environmental fluctuations.

There is no way of predicting how long the response will continue, or how great a total change may be produced by long-continued selection. The experiment illustrated showed an undiminished response for nine generations, which changed the character selected by about 1·8 standard deviations. Experiments continued over longer periods commonly show responses continuing for roughly twenty generations, and producing a total change of some 5–10 standard deviations. We can therefore feel confident that any change that may be taking place as a result of selection in a human population will continue for a long time, provided that the conditions remain the same.

The effect of selection on the variance of the character selected is also unpredictable from theory, because the rate at which the genetic parameters change is not known. In most

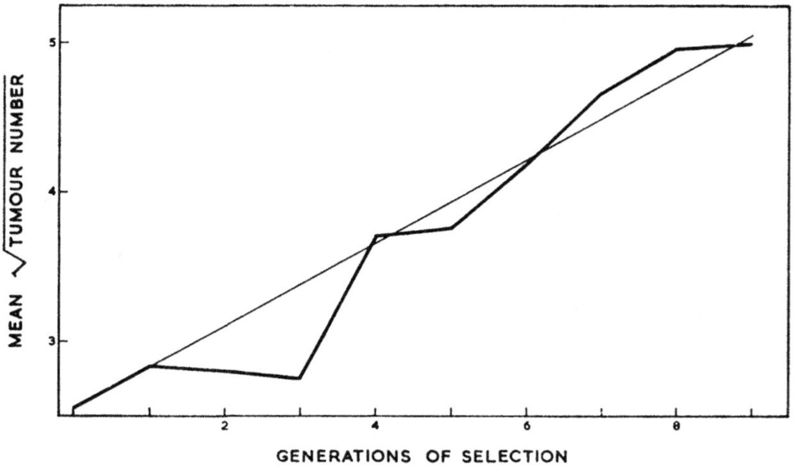

FIGURE 1

OBSERVED AND PREDICTED (THIN LINE) RESPONSES TO SELECTION FOR THE NUMBER OF LUNG TUMOURS INDUCED BY URETHANE IN MICE

The mean of each generation is shown as the mean of the square roots of the individual tumour numbers, the scale transformation being necessary to normalize distribution. (Data from Falconer and Bloom, 1964.[3])

laboratory experiments the phenotypic variance remains substantially unaltered for at least as long as the response continues at an undiminished rate, and when it does change it sometimes increases, even though the additive genetic component has diminished. We can therefore be sure that there will be no large change in the variance of intelligence as a result of differential fertility, though small changes cannot be ruled out.

NATURAL SELECTION

In a laboratory experiment precautions are usually taken to ensure that the environmental circumstances, as they affect the character selected, remain constant from generation to generation, so that no regular change in the mean of the population results from environmental changes. This, of course, is not true of a natural population and we must recognize the possibility—or, in the case of human intelligence, the probability—that the mean value is undergoing a change for environmental reasons. The response to selection predicted by equation (2) is the genetic change, and if there is any environmental change this must be added to give the observed or phenotypic change. In what follows we shall be concerned only with predicting the genetic change in response to natural selection, environmental changes being ignored.

At this point it might be thought that the change of intelligence under natural selection could be predicted from equation (2), since the apparent selection differential could be derived from equation (1) and the heritability of intelligence can be estimated. The prediction, however, is not so simple for the following reason. The 'character' selected under natural selection is not intelligence but 'fitness'; i.e. the individual's contribution of offspring to the next generation. Equation (2) is therefore applicable under natural selection only to fitness, and not to any other character. To predict the change of intelligence we have to consider the behaviour of correlated characters under selection: what change in one character (Y) will result from selection applied to another character (X)? This introduces the concept of genetic correlation.

When we measure two characters in each of a number of individuals and work out the correlation between the two characters, this observed correlation is the 'phenotypic correlation', or the correlation between phenotypic values. It arises, however, from two component causes of correlation, genetic and environmental. A genetic correlation arises when some genes affect both characters (or when genes affecting the two characters segregate in linked combinations, as might happen after recent race-crossing). An environmental correlation arises when some environmental differences affect both characters. The covariance arising from these separate causes are additive to give the observed phenotypic covariance—·

$$cov_P = cov_G + cov_E,$$

whence it can be shown that the three correlations are related as follows:—

$$r_P = r_G h_X h_Y + r_E e_X e_Y, \tag{3}$$

where subscripts P, G, and E refer to the phenotypic, genetic, and environmental correlations respectively, h_X and h_Y are the square roots of the heritabilities of the two characters that are correlated, and $e^2 = 1 - h^2$. The way in which the two underlying correlations, genetic and environmental, combine together to produce the observed, phenotypic, correlation is thus affected by the heritabilities of the two characters. The important point to be noted is that the magnitude of the genetic correlation, or even its sign, cannot be estimated from a knowledge of the phenotypic correlation, even if the two heritabilities are known. A fuller discussion of the relationship between the three correlations is given by Searle.[10]

The genetic change in character Y, when selection is made for character X, can be predicted from the regression equation:

$$R_Y = b_{(G)YX} R_X, \tag{4}$$

where $b_{(G)YX}$ is the genetic regression of Y on X, and R_X is the response of the character directly selected. An equivalent but more informative way of writing the expected change in Y is

$$\frac{R_Y}{\sigma_Y} = r_G h_Y h_X \frac{S_X}{\sigma_X} \tag{5}$$

where σ_Y and σ_X are the phenotypic standard deviations and S_X is the selection differential on X. Thus when the response of Y and the selection differential applied to X are expressed in phenotypic standard deviation units, the response is equal to the selection differential multiplied by the product of the genetic correlation and the square roots of the two heritabilities. So, to predict the correlated response, we need to know the genetic correlation and the heritabilities of both characters, as well as the selection differential. Thus the genetic correlation between intelligence and fitness is of the utmost importance to the prediction of the change of intelligence under natural selection, because there can be no change of intelligence unless there is some degree of genetic correlation between intelligence and fitness; unless, that is to say, there are some genes that affect both intelligence and fitness. It is certainly possible, though perhaps not very likely, that the phenotypic correlation that gives rise to the differential fertility is entirely environmental in origin. There is another important conclusion that is evident from equations (4) and (5), namely that there can be no change in character Y unless character X responds to selection. So intelligence cannot change unless fitness itself changes under natural selection. We must therefore consider the expected change of fitness itself under natural selection.

The expected change of fitness under natural selection can be deduced in the following way. The working is simpler if fitness is expressed as relative fitness, and this simplification does not affect the conclusion. Let f be the number of offspring that an individual contributes to the next generation, and $\bar{f}$ the mean number of offspring contributed by all individuals in the generation. Then the relative fitness, F, of an individual is $f/\bar{f}$. The weighted selection differential is obtained, as explained earlier, by multiplying the superiority of each individual by its relative contribution to the next generation. The character selected and the weight attached to each individual are now the same, namely relative fitness, so the weighted selection differential proves to be simply the phenotypic variance of relative fitness. This can be shown as follows. Putting $f/\bar{f} = F$, and $X = F$ in equation (1), the weighted selection differential on relative fitness becomes

$$
\begin{aligned}
S_F &= \frac{1}{N} \Sigma \left[F(F-\bar{F}) \right] \\
&= \frac{1}{N} \Sigma F^2 - (\bar{F})^2 \\
&= V_{(P)F}. \qquad (6)
\end{aligned}
$$

The expected response of relative fitness, by equation (2) is

$$R_F = h^2_F S_F$$
$$= h^2_F V_{(P)F}$$
$$= V_{(G)F}, \qquad (7)$$

$V_{(G)F}$ being the additive genetic variance of relative fitness. This is Fisher's "Fundamental Theorem of Natural Selection." [4] It is an easy matter to translate from relative fitness, F, back into terms of the absolute fitness, or the actual number of offspring produced, f. The change in absolute fitness, R_f, is related to the change in relative fitness, R_F, by

$$R_f = \bar{f} R_F,$$

where $\bar{f}$ is the mean absolute fitness in the parent generation. The variances of f and F are related by

$$V_f = (\bar{f})^2 V_F.$$

This is true of both genetic and phenotypic components of variance, so the heritabilities of f and F are the same.

The response of any character, Y, other than fitness itself, under natural selection can be deduced from equation (4) as follows:

$$R_Y = b_{(G)YF} R_F$$
$$= \frac{cov_{(G)YF}}{V_{(G)F}} V_{(G)F}$$
$$= cov_{(G)YF}. \qquad (8)$$

Thus the expected change of the character Y is equal to the additive genetic covariance between the character and relative fitness. This result is analogous to Fisher's Fundamental Theorem (equation 7) and might be called the "Extension to Fisher's Fundamental Theorem". It has been stated previously only, as far as I know, by A. Robertson [9] in connection with the improvement of milk yield expected from the selection practised by farmers on the cows in their herds.

INTELLIGENCE AND FERTILITY

As shown by equation (8), the additive genetic covariance between intelligence and relative fitness is the only parameter we need in order to predict the change of intelligence resulting from natural selection. Can this covariance actually be estimated? I am very doubtful if it can, because there are some serious difficulties to be overcome. In the first place, fertility, which we can measure, is not strictly speaking fitness, though I believe it will not matter very much if we assume that it is. If fertility can be accepted as a measure of fitness, then, in principle, the covariance would be estimated in one of two ways—from the component of covariance between groups of relatives in an analysis of covariance, or from the covariance of intelligence in offspring with fertility in parents (or vice versa). There are three main difficulties that I can see: 1, environmental similarity between relatives will lead to an overestimate of the genetic covariance and this will certainly rule out an analysis of covariance based on sibs; 2, the exclusion of individuals with no children will lead to error, and 3, the practical difficulty of measuring both intelligence and fertility in the same individual may render the analysis of covariance impracticable with any sort of relatives. I do not feel competent to make any useful suggestions as to how these difficulties might be overcome.

Though any prediction of the change of intelligence that may be made will require the estimation of the genetic covariance between intelligence and fertility, it is easier to appreciate what are the factors on which a change of intelligence depends, if the prediction is expressed in terms of the genetic correlation, in a manner analogous to equation (5), instead of the covariance as in equation (8). The expected change of intelligence is then

$$R_Y = r_G h_Y h_F \sigma_Y \sigma_F \qquad (9)$$

where r_G is the genetic correlation between intelligence and relative fitness, h_Y and h_F are the square roots of the two heritabilities, and σ_Y and σ_F are the two phenotypic standard deviations.

It may seem surprising that the apparent selection differential on intelligence, which results from the differential fertility, does not appear in the prediction of the response of intelligence. The reason is that the differential fertility is the expression of a phenotypic correlation between intelligence and fertility, whereas the response depends on the genetic correlation. It may, however, be of interest to put the prediction in a form that includes the selection differential, so as to show what proportion of the selection differential is expected to appear as a change of intelligence. It can be shown by a derivation similar to that of equation (8) that the apparent selection differential on intelligence is equal to the phenotypic covariance between intelligence and relative fitness. Thus

$$S_Y = cov_{(P)YF}$$
$$= r_P \sigma_Y \sigma_F$$

whence

$$\sigma_Y \sigma_F = S_Y / r_P.$$

Substitution for $\sigma_Y \sigma_F$ in equation (9) leads to

$$R_Y = S_Y h_Y h_F r_G / r_P \quad (10)$$

In this form the prediction is perhaps rather better adapted to guessing than in any other forms, so let us look more closely at equation (10) and see what value for the genetic change of intelligence might be arrived at by insertion of known or guessed values for the parameters.

The heritability of intelligence is probably the least troublesome factor to estimate. Roberts [8] concludes that something between one-half and three-quarters of the variation in IQ scores is heritable, and Huntley in this Symposium gives the heritability of IQ score as 70 per cent. This is considerably higher than I would have guessed, but, on the grounds that an estimate is better than a guess, I shall adopt it. The value of h_Y is then 0·84.

The heritability of fitness (in the form of its square root, h_F) appears in the equation for the reason stated earlier, that there can be no change of the correlated character (Y) unless the character primarily selected (F) responds to the selection: if the heritability is zero the character will not respond. Now, in the case of fitness, this is the situation that might well be expected in most natural populations. A population subject to natural selection over a long period of time under constant environmental conditions will come to a genetic equilibrium in which fitness is maximal. This is the principle of 'Genetic Homeostasis' developed by Lerner.[6] The heritability of fitness is then zero. A non-zero heritability of fitness will be found only when the population has been comparatively recently subject to a change of environment so that it is now moving toward a new and different genetic equilibrium. This must certainly be true of advanced human populations, because the biological basis of fitness has changed markedly in the very recent past. The number of children in a family is now largely determined by psychological factors in the parents instead of by physiological factors in parents and in children. It will be useless to look primarily for a change in the mean fitness, because it is the genetic change that we need to know and this will be obscured by much larger environmentally caused changes. It may be possible, however, to estimate the heritability of fertility, and this will provide an upper limit to the heritability of fitness itself. In view of the radical change in the biological basis of fitness just mentioned, the heritability of fitness may be quite high—perhaps about 10–20 per cent. I shall take 15 per cent as my guess, which makes $h_F = 0{\cdot}39$.

The last factor to be guessed in equation (10) is the ratio of the genetic to the phenotypic correlation (r_G/r_P), and this is more difficult. The phenotypic correlation can probably be estimated, but it gives no clue to what the genetic correlation may be, as can be seen by consideration of equation (3). The genetic correlation may well be zero, in which case there will be no change of intelligence. Or, the genetic correlation may even be opposite in sign to the phenotypic correlation, in which case intelligence will change in the opposite direction from that indicated by the apparent selection differential. Any guess that we make of the ratio r_G/r_P is dependent on our judgement of the relative importance of genetic and environmental factors as causes of association between intelligence and fertility. If we assume that the degree of association is the same, no matter what the cause of variation is, whether genetic or environmental, then the genetic and environmental correlations will be equal ($r_G = r_E$). On this assumption, and with the values of the two heritabilities known or guessed as above, the ratio r_G/r_P becomes about 1·2. (It may seem surprising that this ratio can exceed one: Searle,[10] explains the conditions under which it can do so.) If we were to assume that the genetic correlation is only one quarter as great as the environmental correlation ($r_G = \frac{1}{4}r_E$), then the ratio r_G/r_P would be about 0·4. The evidence given by Carter in this Symposium suggests that r_G and r_E may not be very different in magnitude, so I shall take 1·2 as my guess of the ratio r_G/r_P.

TABLE I

BAJEMA'S DATA, QUOTED BY CARTER IN THIS SYMPOSIUM, FROM WHICH THE APPARENT SELECTION DIFFERENTIALS WERE CALCULATED

IQ RANGE	NUMBER IN GROUP	MEAN IQ ASSUMED	FERTILITY (actual)	FERTILITY (projected)
≧130	23	136	3·00	2·9
120–129	59	125	2·44	2·4
105–119	282	112	2·24	2·0
95–104	318	100	2·02	1·8
80–94	267	87	2·46	1·6
69–79	30	74	1·50	1·0
Total or mean	979	101·47	2·24	1·84

Inserting these various estimates and guesses in equation (10) gives the expected genetic change of intelligence as ($1{\cdot}2 \times 0{\cdot}84 \times 0{\cdot}39$) S_Y, or about 40 per cent of the apparent selection differential. I think that, if estimates can be obtained to replace the guesses, the change will prove to be less than this. The point I want to emphasize, however, is the difference between natural and artificial selection. If artificial selection were applied to intelligence itself, with a heritability of 70 per cent, the response would be 70 per cent of the selection differential, whereas under natural selection the expected change is 40 per cent, or less, of the apparent selection differential.

Finally, we may look for an estimate of the apparent selection differential, S_Y, itself. Estimates can be obtained from two sets of data quoted by Carter in this Symposium, both referring to populations in the USA. From Carter's tabulations (reproduced in Table I here) I calculated the apparent selection differential to be +0·5 IQ units in the data of Higgins, Reed and Reed, and +0·3 IQ units in the data of Bajema. It seems therefore that the selection arising from the differential fertility in these populations amounts to very little. The expected genetic change going on at the time to which the data refer would, according to the calculations and guesses made above, amount to an increase of one or two tenths of an IQ unit per generation. As Carter points out, however, the spread of family planning into the lower intelligence groups is likely to increase the positive fertility differential. His suggested distribution of family size by intelligence, if all families were planned, leads to an apparent selection differential of 2·1 IQ units. The genetic change might then amount to nearly one unit per generation.

SUMMARY

If differential fertility gives rise to an apparent selection pressure on intelligence, this is an expression of phenotypic correlation between intelligence and fertility. Any genetic change resulting from the selection, however, depends on the genetic correlation, and the phenotypic correlation gives no information about the magnitude or the sign of the genetic correlation. Consequently the genetic change of intelligence cannot be predicted from the apparent selection differential, even if the heritability of intelligence is known.

The predicted genetic change of intelligence in one generation under natural selection is equal to the additive genetic covariance between intelligence and relative fitness. The estimation of this covariance, though possible in principle, may prove impossible in practice.

Alternative forms of the expression for the predicted change, showing more clearly on what it depends, are given in equations (9) and (10). The operative factors are the genetic correlation, the heritability of intelligence, and the heritability of relative fitness. If any of these is zero there can be no genetic change of intelligence. From the estimates available, and some guesses, it seems that the genetic change of intelligence expected from the differential fertility in two surveys may amount to an increase of one or two tenths of an IQ unit per generation. There are, however, grounds for predicting an increase of nearly one unit per generation if the present planning of families were extended to all intelligence levels.

ACKNOWLEDGEMENT

I am much indebted to Dr Alan Robertson for letting me read his paper, and make use of the conclusions in it, before publication.

REFERENCES

1. Crow, J. F. and Kimura, M. 1955. Some genetic problems in natural populations. *Proc. 3rd Berkeley Symp. on Math. Stat. Prob.* **4**, 1.
2. Falconer, D. S. 1960. *Introduction to Quantitative Genetics.* Edinburgh. Oliver and Boyd.
3. Falconer, D. S. and Bloom, J. L. 1964. Changes in susceptibility to urethane-induced lung tumours produced by selective breeding in mice. *Brit. J. Cancer* **18**, 322.
4. Fisher, R. A. 1930. *The Genetical Theory of Natural Selection.* Oxford University Press.
5. Kempthorne, O. 1957. *An Introduction to Genetic Statistics.* New York. Wiley.
6. Lerner, I. M. 1954. *Genetic Homeostasis.* Edinburgh. Oliver and Boyd.
7. Lerner, I. M. 1958. *The Genetic Basis of Selection.* New York. Wiley.
8. Roberts, J. A. F. 1964. Multifactorial inheritance and human disease. In *Progress in Medical Genetics*, Vol. 3. (Ed. A. G. Steinberg and A. G. Bearn.) New York and London. Grune and Stratton.
9. Robertson, A. 1966. A mathematical model of the culling process in dairy cattle. *Anim. Prod.* **8**, 95-108.
10. Searle, S. R. 1961. Phenotypic, genetic and environmental correlations. *Biometrics* **17**, 474.

DIFFERENTIAL FERTILITY AND INTELLIGENCE

Conclusion

J. A. Fraser Roberts

Paediatric Research Unit, Guy's Hospital Medical School, London

I am sure you will agree that this has been a most stimulating afternoon. Four quite splendid papers have followed each other in logical progression. It makes the sort of discussions we used to have in the twenties and thirties look a little naïve. There have been advances in the technique of the collection of information both in its quality and its volume, but it seems to me there have been even greater advances in the technique of analysis. That has been shown very clearly.

I will not refer to the papers in detail, but I am tremendously impressed by Mr Huntley's results. The heart of the great R. A. Fisher would have been delighted, I know, to see a study in which multiple measurements are made on the same subject. It proved most illuminating. Here we see a coherent pattern emerging: in this very difficult field of human measurement here is a sensible pattern with reasonable, rational explanations of what on the whole looks a pretty consistent body of figures. It is instructive to see from Dr Falconer how estimates can be made at the sophisticated level: I hope he will make some more estimates with quite different assumptions as to the pattern of differential fertility. Human populations do not play fair; demographers do their best and produce beautiful projections, and then the unstable behaviour of human beings upsets them all because the changes are so great. It may well be that, given a different set of assumptions, the effect of differential fertility even as short a time ago as, say, fifty years, might have been very different. That is just an incidental thought.

I will not do more now than thank all the speakers at this Symposium, and all who have contributed to the discussions. Let us hope that larger bodies of data and improved methods will tell us even more in the future.

INDEX OF SUBJECTS

INDEX OF AUTHORS

<u>GPSR Compliance</u>

The European Union's (EU) General Product Safety Regulation (GPSR) is a set of rules that requires consumer products to be safe and our obligations to ensure this.

If you have any concerns about our products, you can contact us on ProductSafety@springernature.com

In case Publisher is established outside the EU, the EU authorized representative is:

Springer Nature Customer Service Center GmbH
Europaplatz 3
69115 Heidelberg, Germany

Batch number: 10844623

Printed by Printforce, the Netherlands